Be Fit in No Time

Be Fit in No Time

**TRANSFORM YOUR BODY, MIND, HEART
& SPIRIT WITH MINDFUL MULTITASKING**

R. Makana Risser Chai

ISBN-13: 9781541238510
ISBN-10: 1541238516

Inspirational Hawaii
P. O. Box 846
Aiea, HI 96701
808-282-2743

"I loved this, as it's a wonderful treasure box of exercises, activities and ideas that can be easily incorporated into your 'every day.' This book indirectly challenges the concept of 'Time Poor' and leaves you with no excuses in creating the changes you seek. Loved it!"

--TERESA CORSO

"This book is filled with healing advice. These are great ideas that will improve my physical comfort (I have lots of chronic pain) and emotional well-being. Makana is a wonderful writer and a beautiful woman with loving advice which she is making practical in application for real lives."

-- DR. ALICE BROWN

"Makana gives readers scores of ideas to eliminate time drains and self-sabotaging excuses with 'mindful multitasking,' a new habit one has only to gain from. The fact that she addresses all aspects of one's physical, mental, emotional and spiritual body enhances this book's value. I enthusiastically welcome this book into my wellness regime!"

-- KUMU (TEACHER) BRENDA MOHALAPUA IGNACIO-GORE

Dedicated
to the students of my
"From Stressed to Best" program
for the Financial Education Alliance of Hawaii
who inspired this book
and to
Michael Keolamau Tengan
personal trainer, coach, and friend
who encouraged me to complete it.

Table of Contents

Be Fit in No Time · xiii

Isn't multitasking bad for us? · xvii

Mindful Multitasking is part of a healthy lifestyle · · · · · · · · · · · · · · · xxi

Research supports Mindful Multitasking ·xxiii

Link Mindful Multitasking with your habits · · · · · · · · · · · · · · · · · · · xxv

Physical Fitness ·1

    Breathe deeply ·2

    Tighten your abs ·5

    Use good body mechanics ·7

    Relax your muscles ·10

    Roll your neck & shoulders ·13

    Exercise your face ·15

Extend your back ·······································18

Stretch your hamstrings ································22

Stand up and walk around ····························26

Balance on one foot ··································28

Do squats and lunges ································30

Stretch ··33

Physical Fitness ······································36

Mental Wellness ··37

Relax your mind ·······································38

Listen to positive podcasts, audiobooks, and courses ··········41

Repeat positive affirmations ·························43

Set goals, and assess progress ·······················47

Choose silence ··49

Visualize ··52

Fast every morning ····································55

Mental Wellness ······································57

Emotional Well-Being ··································59

Listen to music ··60

Smile ··62

Sing and chant ·64

Silently sing or chant ·67

Laugh· ·68

Love your work ·71

Be grateful· ·73

Forgive ·76

Love· ·79

Emotional Well-being ·84

Spiritual Being ·85

Experience awe ·86

Listen to guided meditation · · · · · · · · · · · · · · · · · · ·88

Repeat mantras ·90

Meditate ·93

Pray ·95

Listen and watch for answers · · · · · · · · · · · · · · · · · ·97

Spiritual Being ·99

Creating More Time ·101

How to make time ·102

Do what you love ·105

What to do with more time ·107

A Mindful Multitasking Manifesto ·111

Transform Your Life ·113

Thank you – Mahalo ·115

About the Author ·117

Be Fit in No Time

You can be more fit and healthy in body, mind, heart, and spirit without taking any extra time.

It may sound impossible, because we've all been told we have to set aside time to achieve our goals to become healthy and happy. We've all experienced making time to get more fit, and even doing it for a while, then life took over, our schedules got full again, and we had no time to do what we know is best for us.

Or, we're good about setting aside time to get healthy in some ways, yet still don't have time for others. We might exercise and not spend time with family, or spend time with family yet have no spiritual practice.

How many of us have felt regret for not making time to exercise, set goals, do affirmations, practice gratitude, meditate, and pray? Well let me share with you the secret of success. Mindful Multitasking. Do all of those things and more while doing something else you're already doing. If you do this, you'll become healthier and happier in no time.

Although it contradicts conventional wisdom, I've taught Mindful Multitasking to many people who have successfully used it to get fit—sometimes with surprising results. Mindful Multitasking positively affects all aspects of their lives, including work and family. Having used it myself for many years, I know that Mindful Multitasking can transform your life.

Does it still sound too good to be true? If we think that getting fit in body, mind, heart, and spirit takes hours of exercising, reading, journaling, and meditating, then it does sound like a dream. We don't have hours to spend, so we don't do it. Yet if you change your approach, you can become healthy and happy in no time at all.

I started on my path towards healthy living when I was diagnosed with ulcers in kindergarten. I was told that ulcers were caused by stress and that I had to exercise, keep a positive attitude, spend time relaxing, and so on. I joined the swim team in third grade, learned yoga in eighth grade, and started meditating in college.

About ten years ago I became a certified stress and wellness consultant with the Canadian Institute of Stress, founded by Dr. Hans Selye, the physician who discovered in the 1930s how stress impacts our health. I now teach people how to live healthy, happy lives, based on solid, long-term scientific research, my personal practice, and their own experience.

My students often complain they don't have time to exercise, relax, and build their relationships. They work full-time jobs. They have kids. They volunteer. They take classes. On top of that, many of them have chronic pain. They have frequent colds and flu. They're run down and exhausted. For some, it's all they can do to lie on the couch and watch TV.

Yet there are things you can do while lying on the couch watching TV that will make you more fit physically, mentally, emotionally, and spiritually. And the great thing about becoming even a little more fit is that it allows you to do a bit more, which then makes you more fit. That first step easily leads to more steps along your fitness journey.

Mindful Multitasking allows you to practice what you want to do to be healthy and happy. With these techniques that you can do while you're going about your daily routine at home or work, you will become more fit in body, mind, heart, and spirit.

Is spending a few minutes multitasking mindfully as good as spending hours getting fit? Of course not. Yet for many of us, it's better than what we are doing – letting our minds race, and not exercising at all. And if you consistently spend minutes every day practicing these techniques, you will get more healthy and happy and transform your life.

Everyone wants to be more healthy. Even those people who spend an hour a day physically exercising may be worried because they aren't spending time on their mental, emotional, and spiritual well-being. They may fear that their relationships are suffering because of the time they spend exercising. With Mindful Multitasking, their relationships can improve. In fact, you can mindfully multitask while exercising.

Anyone can mindfully multitask. You can do it right now. Right now you can take a deep breath. Inhale deeply. Exhale fully. You can keep inhaling and exhaling deeply while reading this book, or doing anything else at work, at home, or anywhere. Deep breathing has many benefits. It reduces stress, anxiety, depression, and emotional reactions. It increases feelings of calm. Deep breathing helps you think more clearly. It relaxes your muscles, and improves blood pressure, energy, and mood. Imagine having all that while you're just sitting here reading!

Another way you can mindfully multitask right now is to smile. Yes, smile! Research suggests that smiling, even "fake" smiling, changes your brain chemistry and actually makes you happier and more optimistic. Try it right now, and while you read this book.

When you realize how much you can do with Mindful Multitasking, all of the common excuses fade away. Having enough time is no longer an issue. None of these practices requires special equipment. You don't have to join a gym or pay for a class. All you have to do is do it.

The benefits of Mindful Multitasking are that you will feel stronger, work better, live longer, and even look younger. You will be fit in body, mind, heart, and spirit. Your life will be transformed.

Isn't multitasking bad for us?

One day in my law firm, a couple of us attorneys were standing around chatting with staff. I was part of the conversation until the receptionist handed me a letter that had just come in. I stood there, reading the letter. Then I looked up and noticed the conversation had stopped. I didn't think anything of it and walked to my office to deal with the letter. A few minutes later the receptionist came in to complain about an offensive comment one of the attorneys had made during the conversation. She wanted to know why I hadn't said anything. I told her I hadn't heard it. She found it hard to believe, but it was true. I had been multitasking and had completely missed the remark.

My experience is right in line with all of the research that's been done on multitasking. Whether it's checking email during a meeting, talking on the phone while driving, or texting while walking, many studies have shown that multitasking is inefficient, unproductive, and can be downright dangerous. There is an exception, however, and that's where Mindful Multitasking comes in.

The problem with most multitasking is that we're trying to think about two different things at the same time. So we try to write a report while on a conference call, or have a conversation in real life while looking at social media. It doesn't work. You can only think about one thing at a time. Now that makes sense when you think about it. You can't talk and read at the same time. We might think that driving and walking don't take much thinking, and usually they don't, but responding to events on the road do. Research shows that even talking on a cell phone, even hands-free, is as dangerous as drunk driving. Numerous studies have shown that walking while looking at the phone leads to accidents—everything from tripping, running into things, falling off cliffs, and getting hit by cars.

Even when multitasking is not physically dangerous, research suggests it may have bad effects. Studies show that we can lose up to 40% of our productivity when multitasking. It takes longer to finish tasks. We make more errors, which we have to go back to correct. We can't remember what we've done or heard. It interferes with brain processing. We're less creative. Watching TV or reading while eating prevents the brain from processing what we've eaten, so we are more hungry. (On the other hand, good conversation while eating actually helps us digest food better and leads to feeling more full.)

Yet here's the thing about all this research: it's really about "task switching," not true multitasking. When we read email during a meeting, we listen to the meeting, then switch our attention to the email, switch to the meeting, switch to the email, and so on. We're not really doing both at once because we can't think of two things at the same time.

With Mindful Multitasking, you are not thinking of two things at once.

There are actually two types of Mindful Multitasking. One is when you are using the time when you aren't thinking at all. Time spent waiting for the microwave, standing in line, or watching your kids at practice—all of this is time when you have nothing you have to think about. Showering, shaving, putting on makeup, and brushing teeth are so rote we don't have to think while doing them. Most of us waste all this time, by thinking about the past or the future, looking at our phones, or staring into space. Instead, you can use it to get healthy and fit physically, mentally, emotionally, and spiritually.

You can use some of these times to exercise by doing squats, hamstring stretches, or balancing on one foot. You can think of something positive that will lift your spirits and make you feel good. You can meditate or pray, if only for a minute, because you don't have anything else to think about.

The second type of Mindful Multitasking is when you do have to think while doing your normal activity, but what I'm suggesting to do at the same time doesn't take much thinking at all. You can read this book while breathing and smiling. You don't have to think about breathing or smiling once you remember to do them. You can drive while listening to positive audiobooks just as well as you can drive while listening to talk radio. You can cook or clean while playing upbeat music.

Research shows that you can multitask as long as you are not trying to think while doing both activities at the same time. If you are doing something that you've done many times and you're good at, you have freed up your brain to think about something else. We've all experienced this when we've folded laundry while watching TV, or had a deep conversation while going for a walk. That's why Mindful Multitasking works.

Mindful Multitasking is part of a healthy lifestyle

We've all heard that we need some amount of exercise every day. Some studies suggest we need 30 minutes minimum per day, and others find that our health improves if we go up to an hour, five or six days a week (yet it seems no further improvements are found if exercise is done for more than an hour). Then again, it depends on how we define exercise. A real workout brings your heart rate up.

There are some ways you can get a workout with Mindful Multitasking. Squats and lunges can be done while waiting for the coffee maker or tidying the house, and because they work the biggest muscle group in the body, the quadriceps in the front of the thigh, they can get your heart rate up. If you work someplace where you have to go upstairs many times a day, sprinting up the stairs can be a great cardio exercise. If your spouse, partner, or kids practice sports, music, or theater, instead of sitting waiting for them to finish, you can do a full exercise routine.

For most of us, Mindful Multitasking will not be able to replace the 30 to 60 minutes of exercise we need. Nor will a few minutes of meditation give the same amount of benefit as a 20-minute sitting practice.

So why do it? If we aren't exercising or meditating anyway, it's better than nothing. In fact, it's a lot better than nothing, because it gets you started. If all the exercise you ever do is what's in this book, you will be far ahead of where you would have been without it. And as you get stronger, you may find yourself taking a walk, or spending more time standing than sitting, or coming up with your own ways of exercising with Mindful Multitasking.

If you already have an exercise routine, you can look at these techniques as cross-training. Some of them, like balancing on one foot, are often ignored in exercise plans. Others, such as hamstring stretches, are most effective if done every day.

Either way, Mindful Multitasking adds new ways for you to become more strong in body, mind, heart, and spirit.

Research supports Mindful Multitasking

All but one of the techniques in this book are based on solid research. For each technique, I've listed the benefits of practicing it. Every benefit has scientific studies to back it up. Sometimes there is research that supports the technique, and there are other studies that don't. In those cases, I tell you that. In a few instances, I've also given you some warnings about situations where the technique should not be practiced, or recommended you contact your health care provider before trying it.

I am not a scientist. I am a researcher. I made sure that every technique I recommend (except the very last one) has some scientific support. I reviewed hundreds of scientific research papers to come up with these recommendations. Occasionally I cite a study, but I did not list all of the studies or give you footnotes to the research. That would slow down your reading and take me longer to write this book. If you're really interested, you can Google® it as well as I can.

For every technique, I've given you stories about how they have worked in real life. Many times they're about my experience, both successes and "learning opportunities." Please know that I am not perfect. There are days when I forget all this. That's why I teach and write about this—to remind myself.

Sometimes I use stories from friends and students. In those cases, I've changed some of the personal information, or combined two stories into one, to maintain their privacy.

I was speaking to 300 school staffers about these techniques when a woman stood up and asked, "Do you believe this crap you're teaching us?" I was a bit surprised by the question and stammered out, "Yes. Yes, I do believe it." She said, "Well I don't believe it!" I replied, "Thank you for saying that! Because I'm not asking you to believe anything I say. I'm just asking you to consider it. If something sounds good to you, try it. If it works, great. If it doesn't, maybe you can try something else."

That's my advice to you when it comes to everything in this book.

Link Mindful Multitasking with your habits

To make the most of Mindful Multitasking, you will want to make it a habit. One of the best ways to do that is to link it to something else that is already a habit. As you read, decide which technique you want to associate with something you already do. The secret to being successful with Mindful Multitasking is to get into the habit of always doing the technique when you do your regular activity.

For example, every time I brush my teeth I extend my back and do a hamstring stretch. I don't have to think about it, my body just responds naturally. Every time I get in the car in the morning, I cue up the upbeat music so I can sing along. Whenever I use the microwave, I balance on one foot. There are thirty-four techniques altogether, and each one can be paired with something you regularly do.

Here are just some of the things you probably do daily, weekly, or monthly that can be paired with Mindful Multitasking:

- showering
- shaving
- putting on makeup
- brushing teeth
- using the toilet
- driving alone
- driving or riding with family
- riding in public transit

- cooking
- cleaning
- tidying up
- doing laundry
- gardening
- mundane tasks at work (stapling, copying)
- on hold on the phone or online chat
- waiting for downloads or web pages to open
- standing in line
- pumping gas
- exercising
- watching loved ones at practice, game, hobby
- doing your nails
- having your hair done
- waiting for microwave, coffee maker, tea kettle
- sitting in a boring meeting, conversation, speech
- participating in an important meeting or conversation
- walking to or from car or transit
- watching TV
- being on social media
- lying in bed at night

Yes, even when you are lying in bed at night you can practice some of these techniques to feel happy and healthy while you drift off to a good night's sleep. So as you read each one, think about how you could practice it at the same time as something else you regularly do.

In this book, you'll find the thirty-four Mindful Multitasking techniques divided into four sections: physical fitness, mental wellness, emotional well-being, and spiritual being. At the end are some ideas for creating more time in your life, a reminder to use that extra time to do what you love, and suggestions for ways to spend that extra time to become even more happy and healthy.

Just implementing a few of these ideas can transform your life. You will live longer, be stronger, think smarter, feel better, and look younger, all while enjoying life and making the world a better place for all the people you meet.

Physical Fitness

The research is in, and if you want to have a long, healthy, happy life, you want to exercise. Exercise has been found to reduce the risk of cancer, diabetes, Alzheimer's, heart conditions, and pretty much every other chronic disease. It also lifts your mood and prevents or lessens the effect of stress and depression. For many people, exercise is not part of their daily lives. Even if it is, we can always do more.

We've all heard that we can use bits of time to get in the exercise we need. Take the stairs. Park farther away. Stand up when talking on the phone or with others. All of this is good advice, and I highly recommend it. The techniques I'm sharing with you here get your blood moving, increase oxygen in your brain, and build your muscles—all while you're doing something else. Best of all, even though they count as exercise, some of them you can do while sitting in a chair.

Breathe deeply

Deep breathing counts as physical exercise, and it has many of the same benefits. You can reduce stress, anxiety, depression, and emotional reactions. You literally will reduce blood pressure with three breaths. You will increase feelings of calm, and become more clear thinking. Deep breathing relaxes your muscles. And it enhances your energy and mood.

The great thing about deep breathing is that you can do it everywhere always. You can start deep breathing right now, and every time you pick up this book to read.

You might think the last time you would want to multitask mindfully is in an important meeting or conversation, but actually that is one of the best times to breathe. In important meetings and conversations, you have to be fully alert. You need to hear not only all that is being said, but also what is not said, and what is implied. You have to think clearly, not react emotionally, and be ready to respond.

Since deep breathing reduces blood pressure, you feel calmer. It increases the oxygen in your brain, so you think more clearly. By focusing on your breath, you reduce the chatter in your brain. You can concentrate on what others are saying, both verbally and non-verbally.

There are many different ways to practice deep breathing listed below. Perhaps the best way to breathe in an important meeting is to take long slow inhales and exhales silently. No one has to know you're doing it.

Deep breathing is especially useful when we are feeling shocked or upset. Taking a few deep breaths will reduce emotional responses and help you think more clearly.

The first weekend after my husband and I moved to our vintage home, I was cleaning behind the refrigerator and knocked loose a water hose that began leaking all over the floor. I quickly got some towels and stopped the leak for the moment, but in my mind I started catastrophizing. "We have to call a plumber, there will be a huge bill, the whole house is decrepit, we will end up replacing all the plumbing and electric ..." Fortunately, I realized my mind was out of control and started deep breathing. I calmed down, instead of pressuring my husband to come up with an answer fast. Eventually he solved the problem with a $10 part and a little ingenuity. If I hadn't taken the deep breaths, we would have gotten in a fight, I would have called the plumber, and I would have been stressed out the whole time.

How to:
There are many different breathing techniques.

Attention: Simply pay attention to your breath and don't try to change it.

Counting: Breathe in through the nose and out through a relaxed mouth while counting silently. You can breathe in for a count of four, hold your breath for two, and breathe out for six counts.

Affirmations: A variation of the counting method is to replace the numbers with words, such as inhale saying silently to yourself "peace, calm, health, joy," hold and say "relax," exhale with "peace, calm, health, joy, thank you."

Belly breathing: Start with a long slow exhale, then inhale, expanding your belly and chest as much as you can. Hold briefly, then exhale as long as you can, squeezing your belly at the end. This can be combined with positive words, too.

You can find many other techniques looking online, in books, and for classes in meditation, yoga, and pranayama (a yoga breathing practice).

There are also breathing techniques you can combine with visualizations, which we cover in the Visualization section.

Try the various techniques. You may find one more comfortable than another, or one might work better in some situations than others.

You can combine deep breathing with pretty much every other technique. Right now you can breathe and smile, relax your muscles, and feel gratitude.

When to:

Think about something you regularly do where you can benefit from deep breathing. Would it be helpful in an important meeting, when you get upset, or at some other time? You can affirm right now, "The next time I _____, I will take a deep breath."

Tighten your abs

When you have tight abs, it relieves low back pain. Tight abs improve bowel movements, bladder control, and blood circulation. Your posture improves, so you look younger. Your clothes fit better. And it can enhance your sex life.

For years I had chronic low back pain and tried everything—drugs, physical therapy, massage, and yoga. I was a yoga teacher when I heard about Pilates. In my first session I felt like a beached whale. I couldn't do anything! Immediately I signed up for classes, and after eight sessions over three months I lost inches off my waist, and my low back pain was gone forever. Within six months I became a certified instructor, and taught weekly classes for eight years. It was in Pilates that I learned this ab tightening technique.

As to enhancing sex, one of my Pilates students pulled me aside one day and told me her husband said she was tighter now. It was more fun for him, and she admitted, it was more fun for her, too. Other students have said it helped with incontinence and hemorrhoids.

You can tighten your abs pretty much anywhere, anytime. It can be done while sitting, standing, or lying down. You can do it right now. Perhaps a good time to make sure to do it regularly is when you put on makeup or shave, since most of us do that every single day.

How to:

There are two "ends" to tightening your abs. At first, you may need to concentrate on each end separately, but as you get the hang of it, it will become one motion. You can do this right now, as you are reading this.

First, picture a fish hook pulling your belly button back towards your spine and down towards your tailbone.

Second, tighten your pelvic floor, also known as your Kegels. To do this, squeeze your muscles as if you were trying not to pee.

Now put the two together and you are tightening your abs, all your abs: the Transversus Abdominis, Internal and External Obliques, and the Rectus Abdominis.

At first, you can try tightening for 10 seconds, then releasing for 10 seconds, up to a minute. As you increase your muscle tone, go for longer times. Ultimately, you want to keep your abs tight all day—and eventually it can become unconscious and automatic.

People sometimes say, "I can't pull my belly in because the fat is in the way!" Most of the fat is on top of the muscle. We can't pull it in because we've lost muscle tone. But if you keep working it, it will start working.

For even more impact, when you tighten your abs you can tighten your glutes, the muscles in your rear, at the same time. Notice how your posture improves when both abs and glutes are tight.

By the way, when you tighten your abs, don't tighten your face. Smile, breathe, visualize, and affirm, "My abs are tightening."

When to:
Think about something you regularly do where you can multitask by tightening your abs. Is it while putting on makeup or shaving, or another time? You can affirm right now, "The next time I _____, I will tighten my abs."

Use good body mechanics

The way we hold our bodies as we move about in our daily lives can make a huge difference in how we feel. Poor body mechanics are often the cause of pain and injury to the back, neck, shoulders, hips, knees, hands, and feet. Good body mechanics affect how we hold ourselves when we sit, stand, lift, carry, bend, and sleep.

One way to get the benefits of exercise without exercising is to use good body mechanics and posture in your everyday life. Good body mechanics and proper posture work almost all of the muscles in your body, including your abs. Good posture benefits your internal organs, improves circulation, and makes you look younger.

You can use good body mechanics 100% of the time.

How to:

Standing: Stand up straight. Your low back is slightly curved towards your belly, shoulders slide down your torso, chest is lifted. Imagine a golden thread that runs from your tailbone, up your spine and neck, and out through the top of your head. Your neck is long, your chin level. Pull your belly in, and tighten your glutes, the muscles in your rear. If you need to stand for long periods of time, shift your position to increase circulation and relieve your muscles.

Lifting: We all know about using good body mechanics when we lift things off the floor. A good lift includes a good squat, so if you are lifting and lowering a few things, you will get your squats in for the day.

Sitting: If sitting at a desk, your feet should be flat on the floor and the chair low enough that your thighs are parallel to the floor. Although many doctors and chair manufacturers recommend chairs that support your low back, ideally you will sit all day without resting against the back of the chair. (That's what I do, thanks to my Pilates routine.) Get up at least once an hour, walk around, and stretch. If you also are dedicated to staying well hydrated, this can be combined with getting another glass of water.

Driving: Slide your shoulder blades down your torso. Lift your chest. Get even. Is your left foot even with your right? Stretch it out. Is one hip or shoulder higher than the other? Wiggle them to even yourself out. Use a relaxed grip on the steering wheel.

Activities: Use good body mechanics in your activities. When chopping vegetables, working with tools, or sitting at the computer, keep your shoulders level and your chest lifted. While crafting, repairing, or gardening, keep your feet and hips facing the project you're working on, and your hands in front of your body. Don't reach your arms out away from your body unless you absolutely have to. Better to move your feet so that your arms stay in front of your body.

Cleaning: Use the least amount of effort necessary to get a good result. My mother taught me to shake out area rugs by raising them above my head and whipping them towards the ground over and over. Then I realized they get just as clean if I hold my hands at waist level and whip the rug from there.

A doctor once told me to prevent back pain by avoiding one-sided sports. For example, he recommended jogging rather than tennis. Vacuuming, sweeping, and raking are one-sided, but you can make them more balanced. One way is to switch sides, doing half the job using the right arm and half using the left. That's actually good for your brain, too, but might be a little frustrating. Another way to even yourself out is not to face the area you are working, but to turn your side towards it (reversing the advice above since this is one-sided). When vacuuming, for example, I keep my left side towards the area I'm working. Then, depending on my energy level, I use one or two techniques:

(1) I bring both arms far to my right side, pulling the vacuum about even with my left foot, and then push my arms with the vacuum far to the left. The range of motion of my arms is about equal on the right and left sides.

(2) I keep my arms centered in front of me the whole time. I reach out my left foot, and move my entire body to the left, bringing my right

foot and the vacuum with me. Then I reach back with my right foot, bringing my left foot and the vacuum back to where I started. Once you get the hang of it, you'll be dancing. It's kind of a salsa step, and you can get a lot of good exercise doing it.

You can combine good body mechanics with pretty much every other technique. Right now you can sit up straight, feel grateful, and smile.

When to:

Think about something you regularly do where you can benefit from good body mechanics. Is it sitting, standing, or lifting when you could most benefit, or something else? You can affirm right now, "The next time I _____, I will use good body mechanics."

Relax your muscles

We all do it unconsciously, but sometimes we become aware of how much we are tensing our muscles unnecessarily. It could be our faces, necks, shoulders, hands, stomachs, backs, legs, toes, or any other part of our bodies. Research shows that when our muscles are tight, it increases our stress, which then can have negative effects on the body, mind, heart, and spirit.

When you relax your muscles you feel better physically, mentally, emotionally, and spiritually. Relaxing your muscles relieves pain and reduces inflammation, which is associated with many different types of chronic diseases. It also increases your immune function.

We all have seen people who clearly have tense faces or imbalanced shoulders. How often are we aware of our own tension and imbalance? Make a habit of paying attention to your body whenever you are sitting or standing, and relax any tense muscles.

A good time to practice relaxing your muscles is when you are sitting at your computer, waiting, waiting, waiting. You could be waiting for an email, file, or web page to open or download. It could be a few seconds, a minute, or more. Or you can use this technique when you are driving, if you are waiting in backed-up traffic or at a signal.

You also can relax your muscles by not carrying as much. When I practiced law, I carried a briefcase from office to court, but when I went home, I carried a box. Every morning and evening I would carry that box back and forth—yet I rarely actually opened it at night! It was just stuff that I thought I might need. What a relief when I realized I could let go of the box.

What can you let go of to relax your muscles?

This is another technique you can do almost anywhere, anytime. You can do it while you are sitting here reading this book.

How to:

Here are some techniques for relaxing your muscles. You can try some of them right now.

Scan: While sitting, standing, or lying down, mentally scan your body, starting with your feet all the way up to your face. Notice any areas of tension or imbalance (such as one shoulder or hip higher than the other). Release the tension.

Wiggle & Jiggle: While sitting, standing, or lying down, wiggle your toes. Circle your feet, loosening your ankles. Point your toes, stretching your feet, then push out through your heels, stretching your calves. Jiggle your legs. Turn your feet towards each other and away from each other, releasing your hips. Wiggle your hips slightly to improve posture. Stretch your spine up. Wiggle your shoulders up and down. Shake out your arms and hands. Roll your head down and from side to side, stretching your neck. Relax the muscles in your face.

Tense and release: While sitting, standing, or lying down, tense your toes and feet—and then release. Tense your legs—and then release. Tense your abs—and then release. Tense your fingers and hands—and then release. Tense your shoulders—and then release. Tense your face—and then release.

Drop your hands: When driving, relax your shoulders, arms, and hands. Did you know safety experts no longer recommend having the hands on the steering wheel at 10 and 2 as if the wheel was a clock? They now recommend holding them lower, at 9 and 3—which is easier on your arms and shoulders. When the car stops, drop your hands off the wheel completely and let them rest in your lap. Affirm, "I am relaxing." Same thing if you are waiting at the computer for a download or a web page to open.

Let it go: Lighten your load. Think about your briefcase or purse. First, do you really need to carry it at all? Perhaps you can replace it with a backpack which is easier on your shoulders. (When I had a half-mile walk to work every morning, I wore walking shoes, and carried my work shoes and a small purse in a backpack. When I went out to lunch, I took the purse and wore my work shoes.) Second, if you still need a purse or briefcase, can you reduce the weight? Get a smaller, lighter one (leather is heavy), and take out stuff you don't need. Third, pay attention to your body and relax your shoulders. Switch the sides you carry it on so you are even.

Fourth, put it down whenever you can. When you put it down, affirm silently, "I am relaxing now."

You can combine relaxing your muscles with pretty much every other technique. Right now you can relax your muscles, feel grateful, and breathe.

When to:
Think about something you regularly do where you can benefit from relaxing your muscles. Is it working on the computer, driving, carrying, or something else? You can affirm right now, "The next time I _____, I will relax my muscles."

Roll your neck & shoulders

Those of us who spend hours at the computer, on our phones, playing games, watching TV, driving, sitting, or pretty much any other modern activity put stress on our necks and shoulders, which in turn affects our backs. Neck and shoulder rolls are easy to do, and release tension in your face, neck, shoulders, and upper and lower back. They can relieve headaches and improve posture.

This is another technique you can do almost anywhere, anytime. I do these stretches in the car when stopped at lights or in traffic, at the computer while waiting for downloads or chat responses, even in meetings and at church. Back in the late 1970s, I worked for California Assemblyman John Vasconcellos, who was known even in California for his far-out ideas, like the state task force on self-esteem lampooned in Doonesbury. John was criticized in the press for stretching his neck and shoulders while sitting in long committee hearings. I believe it's more socially acceptable now, and even if it's not, the benefits outweigh the risk of criticism.

A good time to do neck and shoulder rolls is while on hold on the phone. Before we talk about that, though, I want to mention what I think is the most important thing you can do for your neck and shoulders when it comes to phones – get a headset. At work, at home, and on your cell, use earbuds or a headset so that you can relax your shoulders and neck. Every time I see someone scrunch a phone between their ear and shoulder, I want to yank it away from them and give them a neck and shoulder massage.

If your work doesn't want to give you a headset, talk to HR and tell them you will get a doctor's note. Or put the phone on speaker so that it annoys all your co-workers and they lobby for you to get a headset. Or just go ahead and buy one with your own funds. It is so worth it.

How to:
You can try some of these right now.

Neck: Turn your head as far as you can comfortably to the right, then to the left. Repeat several times. Drop your head down towards your chest, then look up to the sky, and repeat. Bring your right ear towards your right shoulder, while pulling both shoulders down. Repeat on the left side. Bring your head down towards your chest, and roll your head until the right ear comes to the right shoulder. Roll the head down to center, and up to the left shoulder. (Do not roll your head around to the back, which puts stress on the spine.)

Shoulders: With your head centered, bring both shoulders up towards your ears, and then relax down. Repeat several times. Wiggle your shoulders alternately up and down, first the right, then the left. Then roll your shoulders up, back, down, and around a few times. Lift and expand your chest at the same time. To finish, slide your shoulders down your torso.

You can combine neck and shoulder rolls with many of the other techniques. Right now you can roll your neck and shoulders, smile, and breathe.

When to:
Think about something you regularly do where you can benefit from neck and shoulder rolls. Is it while on the phone, working on the computer, driving, or something else? You can affirm right now, "The next time I _____, I will do neck and shoulder rolls."

Exercise your face

Our faces rarely get much exercise. When you exercise your face, you get all the benefits of exercising your other muscles, and it feels good. The benefit of facial exercise, also called facial yoga, is that it releases tension in the face. It tones the face and neck muscles, and increases circulation, which brightens skin tone. As your face tightens and relaxes with the exercises, you may feel kind of silly, but that's great. If it makes you giggle, even better.

Celebrities have used facial exercises for years with great success. Exercise pioneer Jack LaLanne and actor Richard Chamberlain looked great as they got older, and told interviewers they never used plastic surgery or injections. I happened to sit right next to Richard Chamberlain when he was 82 years old, and his face was beautiful, with no signs of cosmetic procedures. His skin looked elastic, supple, and taut.

This is one of my favorite things to do in the car, especially before an important business meeting or making a speech. I think it's easy for us to allow our faces to freeze into position. This helps your face become more mobile, so that it reflects your feelings and emotions. And honestly, I enjoy it. There is a sense of play, of being a silly kid again.

You can do facial yoga whenever you're alone or don't mind people seeing you make weird faces. It's a good one for when you're on the toilet because no one can see you do it. You may be on the toilet only a few minutes a day, but why not use them in a healthy way?

How to:
You can try some of these right now.

Big yawn: Yawn with a wide, relaxed mouth to release the jaw muscles.

Baby Bird: Tilt your face up. With the tip of the tongue against the roof of the mouth, swallow. Turn your head slightly to the right, and repeat. Then turn to the left, and repeat.

Surprise: Widen your eyes, then squeeze them shut, rapidly shifting from wide to open. Then close your eyes and relax. (If you're driving, just open wide and then relax your eyes, open wide and relax).

Wink: Rapidly squeeze one eye shut, then the other. Repeat.

Wow: Stretch the mouth wide open as if saying, "Wow," showing your teeth, engaging the muscles of the neck.

Smile: Smile as much as you can with a closed mouth, then an open mouth, stretching the lips as far as possible. Raise one corner of the mouth, then the other. If you naturally have one corner that doesn't go as far up as the other, spend extra time on that corner.

Kiss: Stick your lips out with an exaggerated kiss.

O face: Say the letter O, making the opening of your lips as big as possible while still covering your teeth. Bring the corners of the mouth forward and then pull the corners back repeatedly. (Those who know the movie, *Office Space*, may giggle at this name.)

Cheeky: Puff your cheeks out, hold, then release.

Scrunch: Scrunch your face up, then release.

Lion Breath: Inhale through the nose. As you exhale, roar, opening the mouth widely and sticking out the tongue down toward the chin.

Vowels: Say the hard and soft vowels out loud, exaggerating your lips and face. A, ah, E, eh, I, ih, Oh, oo, U, uh.

You can find facial yoga or face exercise videos online as well.

You can combine facial yoga with pretty much every other technique. Right now you can exercise your face, breathe, and think positive.

When to:

Think about something you regularly do where you can benefit from facial yoga. Could it be while using the toilet, driving, or at another time? You can affirm right now, "The next time I _____, I will do facial yoga."

Extend your back

When I taught yoga and Pilates to seniors, they often had two complaints: their low backs hurt, and they weren't as tall as they used to be. In every case, they slumped—they did not extend their backs—and they had tight hamstrings. When our backs are slumped, they are not being used as designed, so they hurt. And when hamstrings are tight, we can't straighten our knees—so of course we're shorter.

The opposite of having a slumped back is to have it extended, that is, your spine curved in towards your belly button. Keeping your back curved inwards relieves low back pain, headaches, tight shoulders, neck pain, and sciatica. It increases circulation. And it improves posture, which makes you look younger.

Tight hamstrings are related to having the back slumped instead of curved and extended. Your hamstrings begin at your pelvis, so if they're tight, they are pulling your pelvis out of alignment which affects your low back. We'll cover hamstrings in the next section.

Most of the time when we sit, we slump with our backs curved out. For many of us, when we stand up we continue to slump. This affects every part of our bodies, internal and external. We've all seen people with their necks bent down and faces almost parallel to the ground. That's what happens ultimately when we slump.

Your body is designed to have your back curved or extended towards your belly button.

You can tell if your back is curved the right way by feeling your lower spine with your hand. You can try It right now. Sit up without resting your back on the chair. When we are curved outwards, our spine pops up and we can feel the joints sticking out. When your spine curves inwards, you can't really feel the joints. Instead, you feel an indentation where your spine is. I call this "your spine in the valley."

You can extend your back pretty much any time you are sitting or standing. My favorite time to do it is when I'm brushing my teeth (combined with a hamstring stretch). That's four minutes a day, and is an excellent way to start and end the day.

How to:

Those who have a herniated disc or scoliosis should not extend the back without first checking with their health care provider.

Standing: (See photos below.) Stand up straight. Feel your spine with your hand and make sure your spine is in the valley. (If it's not, lift and expand your chest, and push your rear end back.) Now bend your knees slightly. Then tilt your pelvis forward, while pushing out your rear. Keeping your back curved towards your belly button, bend your torso slightly forward, hinging at your hips. Lengthen your spine by pushing out through your tailbone and pushing out your rear. Keep your head in line with your spine (don't look up or down), and slide your shoulder blades down your torso. Check your low back with your hand to make sure your spine is in the valley. Many people can only hinge forward a few degrees (photo #1), and that's fine. As you get more practice, you can hinge forward more as in photo #2.

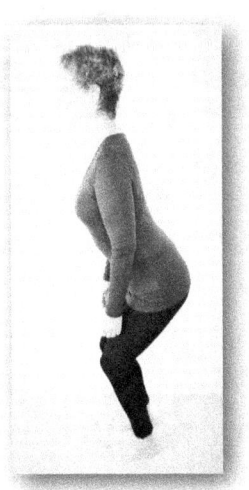
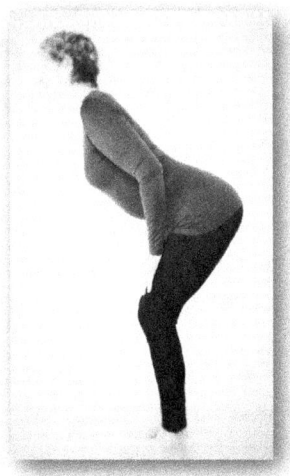
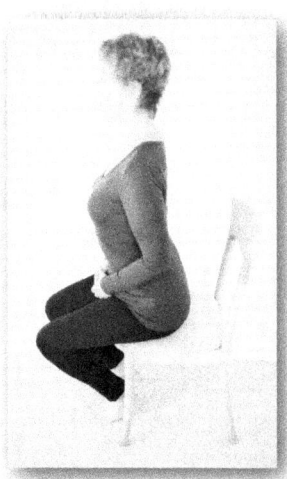

Sitting: (See photo above.) To extend your back while sitting, sit up without resting on the back of your chair. Scoot forward on the seat so your feet are firmly on the ground. Sit up straight. Lift and expand your chest. Tilt your pelvis forward. Slide your shoulder blades down your torso. Check your low back with your hand to feel your spine in the valley. Now stay that way as long as you can.

On the floor: (See photo below.) If you have a moment right now or while watching TV, the best way to fully extend your back is to do the very simple and easy yoga posture called "Cat-Cow." Get down on all fours, with your hands and knees on the floor. First arch your back like a cat. Pull your belly in as you do it. Then reverse the position into cow, allowing your belly and spine (but not your shoulders) to sag towards the floor. Repeat this a few times. It feels SO good! I do it every morning just to get ready for the day.

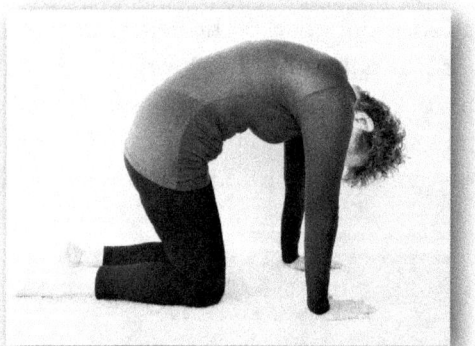 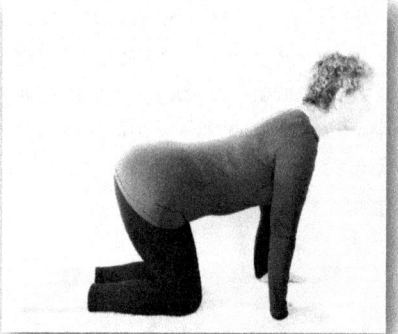

If you have more time: Pilates exercises include extending your back, and the advantage of Pilates is it also strengthens your abs, which helps to support your posture. Research has found that exercises that extend your back have many benefits, including preventing spinal fractures, and increasing bone density in postmenopausal women.

You can combine extending your back with pretty much every other technique, such as smiling and breathing. But it's especially useful to combine it with hamstring stretches, which are next.

When to:

Think about something you regularly do where you can benefit from extending your back. Is it brushing teeth, watching TV, or something else? You can affirm right now, "The next time I _____, I will extend my back."

Stretch your hamstrings

Although athletes pay a lot of attention to their hamstrings, most of the rest of us don't. That can cause problems because the hamstrings are attached to the pelvis, which is the body's center of gravity. From the pelvis, the hamstrings go along the back of the thigh and end just below the knee. When the hamstrings are tight, they pull the pelvis, the center, out of alignment, causing the spine to flatten or slump all the way up to the head. That affects our posture, which in turn strains all the muscles of the back, shoulders, and neck, as well as the internal organs.

The benefits of stretching your hamstrings are reduced pain in the back, knees, and neck, increased knee mobility and hip flexibility, and improved posture. With stretched hamstrings you will enhance daily activities such as sitting, going up and down stairs, lifting, exercising, and bending over.

You can stretch your hamstrings when you are doing other tasks such as standing, sitting on the floor, or lying on the couch, floor, or bed. Stretching your hamstrings one or two minutes a day can achieve great benefits. That's why today I combine my hamstring stretch with extending my back, and do both together while brushing my teeth, but that's not how I started. Many years ago, when I was in yoga school, one of the ways we stretched our hamstrings was through forward bends. We would start like "standing #2" below, then bring our torsos all the way down and rest our hands on the floor. That's what we were supposed to do, anyway. My hands couldn't get past my knees. I decided to practice forward bends for one minute every day, right before I took my shower. Within a year, I could reach the floor.

How to:
Your hamstrings begin at your pelvis and end just below your knee. When your hamstrings are actually stretching, you will feel the stretch behind your knee.

Standing #1: The classic runner's stretch is usually done with hands on a wall or the back of a chair. The front knee is slightly bent, the other leg is stretched behind you, heel on floor, knee straight. You are stretching the hamstring of your back leg, so you should feel a stretch behind your back knee. Keep your hips parallel to the wall or chair. Do not use this stretch if there is pressure on the front knee. This may be a good one to start with if the hamstrings are very tight, but it's not as effective as the ones below.

Standing #2: (See photo #1 below.) This is combined with extending your back (see that section). Your feet are as close together as is comfortable. It starts the same as the standing back extension exercise in the previous section. While extending your back (your "spine in the valley"), bend your torso slightly forward, hinging at your hips, pushing out through your tail. But instead of bending your knees, keep your knees straight but not locked. Feel the stretch behind your knees? That's your hamstrings stretching. We may be able to hinge forward only a few inches—that's fine. This is a good one to do while brushing your teeth, shaving, or putting on makeup.

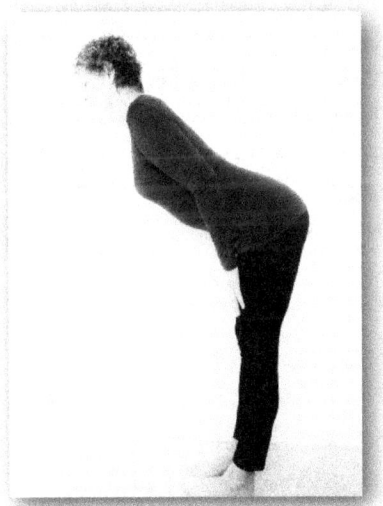 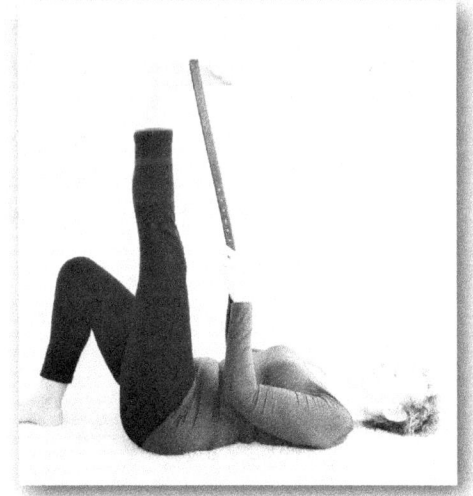

Lying on the couch, floor or bed: (See photo #2 above.) For this, you need something to hold your leg up, such as an old tie, belt, towel, rag, or physical therapy band. Sit down, put the center of the fabric or band around the arch of one foot, holding one end of the band in each hand. Lie down. Bend the knee of your other leg, and put that foot on the couch, floor, or bed. Raise the leg with the band up towards the ceiling. Keep your knee straight, foot parallel to the ceiling, pushing out through your heel towards the ceiling. Keep the weight of your leg in the band so that you are holding it up with your hands. Slide your shoulder blades down your torso and relax your upper body. Keep the band in the arch of your foot—don't put it on your toes and pull your toes, as this can cause injury. Continue the stretch for one or two minutes, then switch legs. You could do this right after you wake up in the morning, before bed at night, or while watching TV.

Sitting on floor: Sit with half of your rear on the edge of a narrow pillow or rolled up towel, so your pelvis is tilted forward. Straighten your legs together in front of you, with your toes pointed towards the ceiling, pushing out through the heels. Bend your torso slightly forward over the straight legs. Visualize your stomach moving towards your thighs keeping your back as straight as possible, rather than rounding the shoulders and the low back. Rest your hands on your legs, sliding your shoulder blades down your torso (photo below). After long practice, perhaps after a year or more, we will be able to bring the elbows to the legs, then the forearms to the calves, and easily touch the toes with the hands. Never reach for the toes, just focus on bringing your elbows to your legs and keeping your upper body straight, not slumped. Feel the stretch behind your knees. This is one you can do while reading, watching TV, or having a conversation.

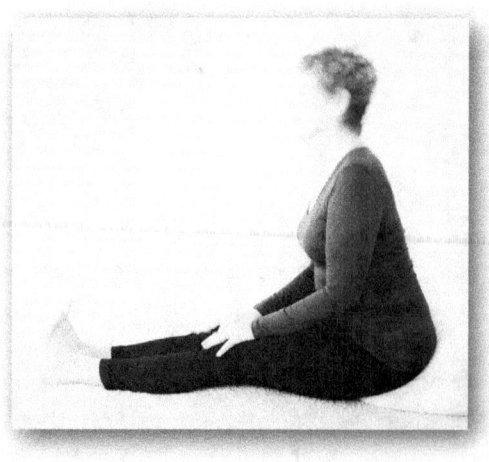

While stretching your hamstrings, you can make affirmations and visualizations that your hamstrings are becoming more flexible. People often say to themselves or aloud, "Wow, my hamstrings are tight!" Instead, say to yourself, "My hamstrings are stretching, releasing, and relaxing." Visualize them softening. Breathe. Love them and be grateful for them. They get you where you're going every day.

When to:

Think about something you regularly do where you can multitask by stretching your hamstrings. Is it brushing teeth, watching TV, or something else? You can affirm right now, "The next time I _____, I will stretch my hamstrings."

Stand up and walk around

As an attorney who has investigated disputes in the workplace, I can't tell you the number of problems that have been caused or made worse by email. I remember one department of five people whose cubicles were next to each other, but no one ever talked. Instead, they sent email flames all day. Even when people in the workplace do talk to each other occasionally, many times emails are misunderstood and lead to disputes and hurt feelings.

On top of that, sitting in the cube or office all day sending emails is not healthy for us physically, mentally, emotionally, or spiritually. For that reason, I'm suggesting that you respond to some emails by standing up, walking to the other person's desk, and standing there to have a conversation.

The benefits of walking and standing are obvious. It gets your blood circulating, and increases the oxygen in your brain, so you think more clearly. Standing—especially with good posture, proper body mechanics, and tight abs—is an exercise in itself. And having a conversation with someone in person engages the brain and nervous system to increase our feelings of well-being. Good relationships with others are essential for emotional health.

Of course, there are lots of other times and places to stand up and walk around, both at work and home. Get up every hour to get a glass of water to drink, and you will stay well hydrated. Get up to talk to a family member, rather than yelling from across the room. Or get up, stand up, and walk outside around the office or house, just to get a breath of fresh air.

How to:
There are at least four times when it is worthwhile to respond to an email by standing, walking, and having a conversation in person. One is where the email involves a rather complicated issue that would most easily be resolved by talking. Another is where one or the other person is offended or upset. Third is when we receive an email from someone we haven't talked with for a while and we just need to touch base. And fourth is when we are

feeling bored or tired and need to take a break. When I was working in an office, I did this almost every afternoon.

When to:

Think about something you regularly do where you can multitask by standing and walking around. Is it to respond to emails, drink water, or something else? You can affirm right now, "The next time I _____, I will stand up and walk around."

Balance on one foot

Balancing improves coordination, burns calories, and stabilizes your hips. It improves your posture, as well as your form for exercise. It strengthens the muscles of the abs, hips, thighs, glutes, and low back. Most importantly, especially as we get older, it prevents falls.

I was in the parking lot of a big box store, moving my new printer from the cart into the trunk of my car. As I picked up the large carton, my shoe caught in a small pothole, and I started to fall. Yet I quickly regained my balance and managed to let down the printer without falling. I firmly believe the disaster was averted due to my practice of balancing.

You can multitask by balancing on one foot any time you are standing. I was once waiting in the kitchen for the microwave and started wondering how many minutes I had stood in how many kitchens waiting for tea kettles, coffee makers, and toasters. It's only a minute or two each time, but even in one day that might end up to be five or ten minutes. Multiply that by your lifetime, and you have a lot of time to balance.

How to:

Balancing on one foot is best done barefoot or wearing flat shoes. Bring your weight onto one leg, slightly bend the knee of your other leg, and bring that foot either slightly forward or back, keeping your hips level. You can lift your foot a quarter inch or more. Squeeze the butt muscle of the leg you're standing on. Lift your torso away from your hips. Relax your shoulders and face. Hold for thirty seconds or one minute, then switch legs.

If at first it is hard to balance, hold on to a wall, chair, counter, or desk. Eventually, support yourself with one finger, and then go hands-free.

To make it more difficult—and get more benefits—you can bring your free leg far out to your side, further out behind you, swing it front to back, or bend your knee towards your chest. You can bend your leg behind you and hold on to your ankle (photo below), which also is a great stretch for the quad muscles in your thighs (especially important if you've been doing squats and lunges). You also can close your eyes—but only after you've mastered balancing for at least a minute with eyes open.

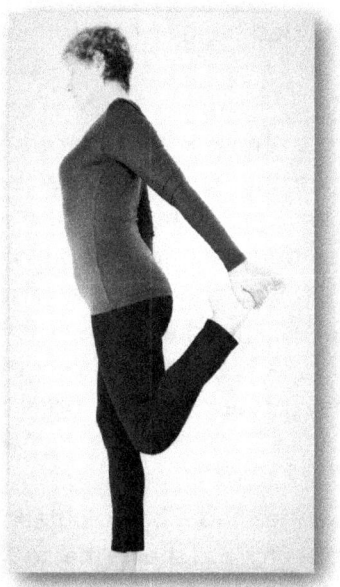

It is more effective to balance one minute every day than several minutes once a week.

You can combine balancing on one foot with pretty much every other technique. You can affirm, "I am balanced" and visualize that applying to all parts of your life. You can breathe, smile, say a mantra, pray, or think loving thoughts at the same time.

When to:
Think about something you regularly do where you can multitask by balancing on one foot. Is it while waiting in the kitchen, standing in line, or something else? You can affirm right now, "The next time I _____, I will balance on one foot."

Do squats and lunges

Exercise great Jack LaLanne said that if you can do squats, you will always be able to get on and off the toilet. When I mentioned that to my then 80-year-old mom, she added them to her morning exercise routine. She's still doing them at 90.

Squats are an amazing exercise with a lot of benefits. Lunges are sort of half squats and have the same benefits. Both squats and lunges work the largest muscle group in the body, the quads in the front of the thighs. Strong muscles burn calories, so building the biggest muscle burns the most calories. Squats and lunges also strengthen your hips, glutes, hamstrings, calves, knees, and abs. They enhance mobility, balance, and coordination. A regular practice of squats and lunges can prevent falls. And they protect against obesity, diabetes, and heart disease.

For years, squats and lunges had a bad reputation for being hard on the knees. More recently, research has shown that they actually strengthen the muscles around the knee, and do not have a negative impact on joints—as long as they're done correctly. That's why it's important to keep proper form. The muscles around the knees may feel sore the next day, but that means you are building them up. If there are concerns about the knees, talk with your health care provider, personal trainer, physical therapist, or exercise physiologist to make sure you are using the right form.

I've been doing squats and lunges three to four times a week for several years now. I don't hate them now as much as I used to. They do get easier.

A great time to multitask doing squats and lunges is when you're tidying the house, garage, or office. Tidying almost always involves picking up things from the floor. Rather than bending over, which can stress the back, use the opportunity to do squats and lunges. You also can do them while waiting in the kitchen, talking on the phone, or other times you are, or could be, standing around. A great ad from Kaiser

Permanente shows a dad and mom doing squats while pushing their kids on swings.

How to:

Squats: Stand with your feet a little more than shoulder width apart, feet pointed forward or slightly outwards. Stand tall, chest lifted and expanded. Keep your back extended (curved inward with your "spine in the valley" as explained in the section on extending your back). Do not allow the spine to slump outward. Slowly bend your knees, and lower yourself as if you were going to sit down in a chair. Keep your rear end pushing back. Do not tuck your tail. Your knees stay over your feet. Keep lowering. Ideally, your upper legs will come parallel to the floor, but you may have to work up to that. Just go as far down as you can. Hold for one to ten seconds. As you move down, you also can bring your arms up straight parallel to the ground for balance. Stand up. Repeat. Breathe in as you go down, breathe out as you go up.

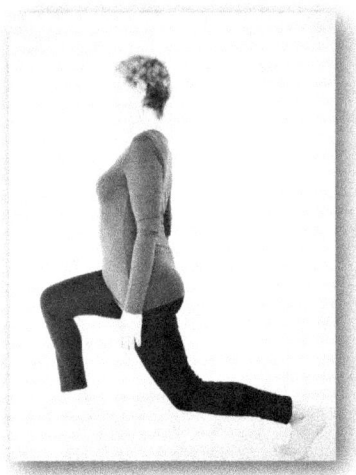

Lunges: (Photo above.) Stand with your legs comfortably together. Step your right foot forward as far as you can. Bend your back knee towards the floor, bending your front knee at the same time, with the goal of your thigh becoming parallel to the floor (this may take some months of practice, just do what you can). Your back foot is up on your toes. Hold for a few seconds or more, then switch sides. Repeat.

If squats and lunges are new to you, take it easy. Start with three or four, every other day. We may feel the muscles ache the next day. That's normal. As we keep doing them, the muscle ache will go away. That means your muscles are stronger. But, again, if you're concerned, seek professional help.

You can combine doing squats and lunges with pretty much every other technique. While doing squats you can smile, visualize, affirm, or pray.

When to:
Think about something you regularly do where you can multitask by doing squats and lunges. Is it while tidying the home or garage, gardening, or another time? You can affirm right now, "The next time I _____, I will do squats and lunges."

Stretch

Stretching improves your posture and physical performance. It enhances coordination and prevents injuries. Stretching releases mental and muscle tension, and increases energy, flexibility, range of motion, and circulation. Stretching also calms your mind.

You can do stretching while standing, sitting, or lying down. I stretch almost every time I stand up at home or in the office, usually for just 5 or 10 seconds. One of my favorite places to stretch is on long plane trips. I usually can find a place to stretch next to an exit door or galley area. If not, I will stretch in my seat. Yes, my seatmates give me weird looks, but I think they secretly wish they could do it too.

For eight years, I taught Pilates and yoga two days a week at the county parks and recreation gym. For the past three years, I've been taking boxing classes three times a week at another parks and rec gym. I love being surrounded by all the active kids and adults. At any given time there are people working out in the weight room, playing basketball, baseball, football, volleyball, and soccer, swimming or running laps, and taking exercise or dance classes, not to mention the little kids running around and playing on the jungle gym.

And then there are their grandparents, parents, spouses, partners, siblings, and kids, sitting in the stands, most of them staring at their phones. Week after week, month after month, they sit there. And I have to admit, I just want to shake them and say, "Get up! DO something!"

I see the same thing at the dance studio near my job, with friends whose kids are in music classes, and with a neighbor who sits and watches her husband work on the car.

If you are a sitter, get up and stretch!

Then after you stretch, you can walk, jog, do jumping jacks, lunges, squats, or anything else to keep moving. Bring an exercise mat so you can do floor exercises like push-ups and sit-ups. Is there an exercise class going on at the same time? Join it. Not sure what to do? You can find yoga, stretching, and calisthenics videos on your phone to follow along. By the way, you can invite your fellow watchers to join you and get even more benefits.

Or you can just stretch.

How to:

Standing: Reach both arms up and stretch to the ceiling or sky. Alternate stretching one arm slightly higher than the other. Feel the stretch in your ribs and out of your hips. Grasp your left wrist with your right hand, pull the wrist towards the right, sticking out your left hip to the left. Repeat on the opposite side. Bring your arms down and slide your shoulder blades down your torso.

Twist: With your feet about hip's width apart, hold your arms out to the right and left, at shoulder height, parallel to the floor, in a T position. Twist your torso to the right, then to the left, and repeat. Or with your arms relaxed at your side, twist to the right and left, allowing your arms to swing like heavy ropes.

Standing forward bend: If you know yoga, or can take a yoga class or watch a video to learn the basics, you can do a simple forward bend. Stand with your feet as close together as comfortable. Hinging at your hips, sticking out your rear, bring your torso down over your thighs. Rest your hands on your legs or the floor. Hold for a few seconds, up to a minute. To come back up, bend your knees, rest your hands on your legs, and roll up, rounding your back, keeping your hands sliding up your legs rather than hanging down loose. This method of coming up (which is different from what most yoga teachers show) will protect the low back from injury.

Sitting: You can do almost the same as the standing stretch when you are seated. Reach up with your arms. Alternately reach one higher than the other. Grasp one wrist and pull it over your head to the opposite side.

Lying down: Bring both arms overhead so they rest on the floor or bed. Stretch your right side, from fingers to toes, then stretch the left side. Stretch diagonally—the right arm and the left leg at the same time, then the left arm and right leg.

You can combine stretching with pretty much every other technique, including neck and shoulder rolls, squats, breathing, smiling, loving, gratitude, and affirmations.

When to:
Think about something you regularly do where you can multitask by stretching. Is it when you get up from your chair, while watching a loved one at practice, or another time? You can affirm right now, "The next time I _____, I will stretch."

Physical Fitness

Here are the twelve techniques for increasing your physical fitness:

Breathe deeply
Tighten your abs
Use good body mechanics
Relax your muscles
Roll your neck & shoulders
Exercise your face
Extend your back
Stretch your hamstrings
Stand up and walk around
Balance on one foot
Do squats and lunges
Stretch

Consider adding them to your daily routine. And if you can think of other physical exercises you can do with Mindful Multitasking, add them in, too.

Mental Wellness

So far we've focused on physical techniques for Mindful Multitasking. Now let's look at mental aspects. The idea here is to both relax and energize your mind. Relax so that the mind is not racing, worrying, or stressing. Energize by replacing negative thoughts with positive ones. Your thoughts can make you feel healthy not only mentally, but also physically, emotionally, and spiritually.

Relax your mind

Worry causes stress. Stress can lead to chronic illness and disease. It can cause panic attacks. Worry makes it harder to think clearly and can result in making bad decisions.

So relax your mind. Be happy and relaxed no matter what. This is called emotional control.

Many of us are familiar with the Serenity Prayer: "God grant me the serenity to accept the things I cannot change, the courage to change the things I can, and the wisdom to know the difference." A few days ago I was repeating this prayer over and over while walking in the woods. It occurred to me that 99.99% of everything in my life falls into the first category, "things I cannot change." The only things that I can change are things I think and do—and even those are not easy to change when they are habits.

If a problem is out of your control, don't worry about it—accept it. Don't get upset—ignore it. Don't complain—pray. Or as the Buddhist proverb puts it, "If you have a problem that can be fixed, then there is no use in worrying. If you have a problem that cannot be fixed, then there is no use in worrying."

I once spent a solid month trying to decide which job I would take, and then only got one offer.

Interpret things in the best way possible until proven otherwise. Not long ago my husband got a text from the woman who recently had bought our house. She wanted to know our address so she could send us a letter. He immediately assumed there was a problem with the house and she wanted us to give her money to fix it. I looked at the text and assumed that a letter had arrived at the house instead of being forwarded by the post office. I was right. But even if I was wrong, at least I would have had two fewer weeks of worry.

It doesn't matter what happens to you. You can choose your response. For eight years I regularly attended weekend retreats. We all slept together in a rough dormitory, with crying babies, loud snorers, wild weather, and a thousand other things that kept me from sleeping. When I finally got up, I would be irritable for the rest of the day because I hadn't slept. But one morning I realized I did not have to be grumpy just because I didn't sleep. I could choose to have a good day! At least that way I wouldn't have a bad night *and* a bad day.

Relax your mind by changing your relationship with the news. I believe it is good to know what's going on, but we may need to put limits on it to preserve our mental health. Watching news on video can sear terrible images into our brains that can come up again at any time. Photos may be less terrifying, and text even less. When we watch TV news or hear it on the radio, it comes at us whether we want it or not. We don't know what's coming next. If we get the news online or in a newspaper, we can quickly skim the headlines, read up on what interests us, and let go of the rest.

Years ago, my boyfriend and I had made a date to walk in the woods on September 11. That morning at 4:30, a friend called and said, "Go turn on the news! A plane hit the World Trade Center!" I got up immediately but did not turn on the news. Instead, I prayed and meditated for an hour. I prayed for the victims, their families, and for the first responders and their families. I didn't know any specifics, but I knew enough. Later, I drove to my boyfriend's house to keep our date. He had been watching the news non-stop all morning. He said, "We can't go hiking now! We have to watch the news." I said, "You are not doing anyone any good watching the news, and you are freaking yourself out. Let's go walk in the woods and pray." And so we did. To this day, I have only once glimpsed a video of the disaster. I have prayed many, many times over. I know this is healthier for me, and I believe it was of more real help to the people involved.

Of course, if we are personally affected by a disaster, our responses will be different. As we grieve, we may feel the need to revisit the events over again. Some who lost family in 9/11 have gone on to dedicate their lives to keeping the memory alive, which has given them peace in their grief. Grieving is its own process for each person. We may be able to use some of the techniques in this book, including relaxing the mind, to ease us through our grieving.

Another way to relax your mind is to focus it. It is so easy for us to allow our minds to wander into worry. If you focus on what you are doing, you do a better job, and your mind relaxes. If you are in a meeting, listening to a speech or sermon, or taking a class, repeat in your mind what the speaker is saying to reinforce the message. This technique compels you to pay attention, and both focuses and relaxes your mind.

How to:
When we find ourselves worrying, we need to replace those thoughts with relaxing thoughts. Telling ourselves not to worry doesn't work. Dr. Norman Vincent Peale suggested visualizing that you are flushing out the worrying thoughts. An ancient native Hawaiian technique I have used successfully is to "oki" or cut off the thoughts. I visualize my arm sweeping down from ceiling to floor in a cutting motion while I say to myself, "I cut off those thoughts."

Then replace the worry thoughts with relaxing thoughts. Think about the last time you were in nature, a fun event you're planning, something that made you laugh or feel loved. Think about your pet or your loved ones. Repeat the relaxing thoughts over and over and over.

You can combine relaxing your mind with many of the other techniques, such as breathing, smiling, listening to music, singing, and more.

When to:
Think about the times you worry. Is there any pattern to them? Do they happen when you are doing certain things? Affirm, "The next time I worry I will relax my mind."

Listen to positive podcasts, audiobooks, and courses

Listening to self-help and spiritual books, courses, and podcasts increases mental stimulation, keeping the brain sharp. They can enhance your mood, and increase feelings of inner peace, empathy, and tranquility. Positive messages can decrease feelings of depression. As you relax and reduce stress, you will lower your blood pressure. Positive messages open the heart and stir the soul.

Listening to positive messages—instead of news and talk radio—while doing chores, driving, or traveling on a bus, train, or plane, can make a huge difference in your day.

If you currently listen to the news or talk radio, I can relate, because that's what I used to do, too. I believe it is good to know what's going on, yet we may need to put limits on it. I used to listen to news on National Public Radio or AM talk radio driving in to work every morning. No wonder I would arrive depressed! These days I get most news online or in a newspaper. You can quickly skim the headlines, read up on what interests you, and let go of the rest.

If you are listening to self-help, educational, or inspirational content, listening with the whole family can help you support each other in living up to the ideas you hear. It's also a good way to start deep conversations with your spouse, partner, or children.

One of my favorite tapes, back in the day when we had tapes, was an hour-long speech by the Rev. Dr. Norman Vincent Peale. I listened to it about once a month for years, and to this day can quote it to you. I always think of a story he told about problems. He concluded, "The only people who don't have problems are dead! So it follows the more problems you have, the more alive you are!" That bit of wisdom still helps me today.

How to:

There are lots of different genres to listen to. Find ones that fill your mind with positive thoughts, thoughts that will stay with you throughout the day, the week, and the rest of your life. Although it can be fun to escape into a novel or adventure, balance it with programming that will help you be healthy and happy.

If there are self-help or spiritual authors you've enjoyed in the past, try their audiobooks. When you find one you like, check online to see what other people who liked that also bought.

One podcast that consistently inspires me is the TED Radio Hour on National Public Radio. No matter how uninspiring the titles of each segment, I almost always learn something I can apply that day to improve my life.

You can combine listening to positive messages with many other techniques, including breathing, smiling, loving, gratitude, visualizations, and affirmations.

When to:

Think about something you regularly do where you can multitask by listening to positive messages. Is it while driving, doing chores, or some other time? You can affirm right now, "The next time I _____, I will listen to positive messages."

Repeat positive affirmations

Affirmations are positive statements about yourself. There are at least three different kinds. One is where you visualize yourself successfully performing—in work, sports, music, theater, or elsewhere—which we cover later under Visualizations. Another type is affirming something that does not exist—for example, saying "I am wealthy" when it's not presently true. We cover that in Visualizations, too.

Here we are talking about affirmations that remind you of something that is presently true for you. If you say, "I am lucky" or "I am blessed," it is true because you are alive, you can think, and you can say those words. You have lots of other reasons to feel lucky or blessed. We often forget about those reasons because we focus on our problems. Affirmations move your focus to the positive.

The benefits of affirmations are that they increase optimism, and put negative events in perspective. They help you focus on what you want to increase in your life. Positive affirmations improve energy and mood. Research with top athletes has shown that affirmations can increase muscle strength and performance.

Do positive affirmations really work? A lot of people claim they do, although scientific research suggests the answer is, "It depends." Try them and see if they work for you.

One of the great old motivational speakers (whose name I've forgotten and haven't been able to find) used to say that whenever something bad happens, affirm over and over again, "This is WONderful!" Years ago, my law partner announced she was leaving the firm. I was devastated. I hadn't even wanted to start a law firm, but she had persuaded me to go in with her. As I drove home that evening, my mind raced with negative thoughts. Then I remembered this advice and started saying, "This is WONderful! This is WONderful!" At first, I could barely say it through my tears, but by the time I got home I realized, it was wonderful! I hadn't been happy in the partnership and now I could get out.

Bhagwan Shri Rajneesh (or Osho) taught that whenever we experience illness or disability, we should affirm, "This illness is a blessing." How many times have we been burned out and then got sick? It was as if Spirit was forcing us to stop. Not long ago, I injured my back moving boxes, and the doctor advised long walks in flat areas. It was a blessing to spend several weeks in daily walks exploring new neighborhoods.

You can say affirmations silently to yourself pretty much anywhere, anytime, and you can say them out loud. I like to say them first thing in the morning, last thing at night, and at meals.

You can make affirmations as a family, perhaps while driving together. Maybe each person can pick one affirmation that everybody says four times.

Another favorite time for affirmations is during exercise, because it allows you to exercise your mind as well as your body. I don't know about you, but when I exercised I had a tendency to make negative affirmations. "This is too hard." "I don't think I can finish this set." "I'm not strong enough to lift this weight." All of these and more had gone through my mind. One day I was struggling with the weight the trainer had placed on the machine. All of a sudden a Bible verse came to me, "I can do all things through Christ who strengthens me." (Philippians 4:13) Suddenly, I was able to lift the weights easily. My trainer said, "Wow! You're working it! Let's increase the weight next set." Which is good, right?

Since then, I make it a point to make positive affirmations to myself. "I can handle this." "I am strong and getting stronger." "Just 30 more seconds."

Affirmations during exercise don't have to be limited to ones about the exercise itself. You can repeat any positive affirmations. And you can use affirmations at any other time.

In fact, you can repeat positive affirmations whenever you are doing something less than pleasant. If you are on hold on the phone with customer service, or waiting for customer service chat responses online, make affirmations. Instead of affirming your impatience and asking yourself over and over, "Why is this taking so long?!?!?!" you can say to yourself "I am peaceful," "I am calm." "I am enjoying this break in my day." "I will be pleasant whether or not I get what I want." "I will treat the other person with love and respect."

How to:
Here are some examples of positive affirmations:

I am grateful (for my home, my job, my health…)

I love (myself, my spouse, my children, my co-workers …)

I forgive (myself, my spouse, my children, my co-workers …)

I trust (myself, God, Higher Power, Spirit)

I am relaxing now

I am strong

I am full of joy

I am patient

If you are a person of faith, you may want to use phrases from a religious text. "A righteous man falls down seven times and gets up." (King Solomon in Proverbs, 24:16) "My mind is unshakable. Words of hatred and anger shall not pass my lips." (Teachings of Buddha) "E ala, e hoa i ka malo. Get up and gird your loincloth. A call to rise and get to work." (Hawaiian Proverbs 259) I believe every religious and spiritual tradition has positive affirmations you can use for inspiration.

Sometimes you may want to affirm something that is true, yet hard to believe. If we're sick, the subconscious will resist us if we say, "I am healthy."

Instead, you can say, "I am getting healthier every day," or "I am taking care of my health."

Repeat your affirmations over and over and over, silently or out loud.

You can combine affirmations with many other techniques, including breathing, smiling, visualizations, prayer, and awe.

When to:
Think about something you regularly do where you can multitask by repeating affirmations. Could it be first thing in the morning, at night before bed, while exercising, or at some other time? You can affirm right now, "The next time I _____, I will repeat affirmations."

Set goals, and assess progress

The benefits of setting goals are well documented. Setting goals increases mental focus, performance, and effectiveness. Goals enhance your feelings of purpose, achievement, well-being, happiness, satisfaction, and success. Goals prevent us from getting bored with life. At work, setting and achieving goals may lead to recognition, promotions, and raises.

In an academic article, Gary Latham and Edwin Locke wrote, "more than 1,000 studies conducted by behavioral scientists on more than 88 different tasks, involving more than 40,000 male and female participants in Asia, Australia, Europe and North America, show that specific high goals are effective in significantly increasing a person's performance."

Or, as baseball great Yogi Berra put it, "If you don't know where you are going, you might wind up someplace else."

Latham and Locke also discuss pitfalls, one of which is that having goals may create stress. I have written five books, including this one. The first was due under a three-year contract, and the third I wanted out by the date of a conference. The second and fourth books I just decided to work on as the spirit moved; one of those took eight years! I've found that although there is stress with goals, at least the work gets done. Without goals, there is stress because the work hangs over my head until it's done.

You can set goals and assess your progress against goals almost anywhere, anytime. It's most effective if you do it on a regular basis, so connecting goal setting with something else you regularly do is a good idea.

Typically we may think of goal-setting as a writing exercise done while sitting quietly. Though that's a great way to set goals, it's not the only way. You can think right now of a goal that is difficult but important to you, visualize it, set a date, and start working on it.

When you are doing or having your nails done or hair cut, you can focus on improving yourself more than superficially. Once your goals are set, the next time you have hair or nails done you can assess your progress on the goals. Do this consistently, and you will meet your goals.

Another time to set goals is when driving with the family. Each person can say what their goals are for the family, and for themselves. In later trips, remind each other of your goals, and assess your progress.

How to:
You may have heard of SMART goals: Specific, Measurable, Attainable, Realistic, Time-bound. Another concept is HARD goals: Heartfelt, Animated, Required, Difficult. And there are many other approaches.

Good goals are:

important to you,

difficult but not impossible to achieve,

easy to visualize what achievement looks like,

to be achieved by a certain date, and

worked on almost every day.

You can combine goal setting with many other techniques, including breathing, smiling, and relaxing your muscles.

When to:
Think about something you regularly do where you can multitask by set-ting goals. Could it be while having your hair cut or nails done, or some other time? You can affirm right now, "The next time I _____, I will set my goals."

Choose silence

Over time, excessive noise causes stress. Whether from neighbors, roads, air traffic, kids, television, music, or anything else, it can affect our memory and emotions. Noise has been linked to high blood pressure, lack of sleep, heart disease, and tinnitus (ringing in the ears). Even white noise, which is supposed to be soothing, can cause stress, distraction, and lack of concentration and focus if it's too loud. White noise is better than excessive noise, but silence is best.

Silence reduces stress, lowers blood pressure, improves memory, and lifts emotions. Research suggests that silence actually may help grow new brain cells, preventing dementia and depression. Silence creates deep relaxation.

The first time some friends visited my apartment, they were excited about how "zen" it was. "It's so peaceful and quiet!" they exclaimed. I excused myself for a few minutes. By the time I got back, they had turned on both the stereo and the TV! For those of us used to living in a noisy environment, it may be difficult to get comfortable with silence at first. Yet it can be done!

How to:
At work: We may work in a place where nothing can be done about the noise. If so, breathe, smile, and use some of the other ideas in this book to counteract the stress it may be causing. Perhaps you can wear earplugs or noise-canceling headphones to reduce the noise level. Consider going to a quiet place during lunch and breaks to give yourself relief.

With some thought, you may be able to find ways to decrease noise in your environment. In one office, they moved the enormous, loud paper shredder from the workspace to the back room. Employees in the cubicles got together and agreed to use ear buds when listening to music or watching videos on their computers. They also stopped yelling across the room to get the attention of co-workers and instead walked over to have conversations.

At home: Make your home an oasis of silence as much as you can. Don't use the television, radio, or music as constant background, and instead choose silence. Talk softly. If you want to say something to someone in another room, get up and go talk to them (which is good exercise), rather than yelling across the house. Close doors gently. Turn off the clicking and beeping noises on your devices, and ask your family to do the same. Close doors on kids, spouse, or partner who are making noise. Ask them to turn off the sound on their devices when they're with you, or use ear buds. You can buy wireless headsets for TVs so that only those watching can hear them. If your dog barks incessantly, figure out why and solve the problem. (Your dog—and your neighbors—will be grateful.) We may think we're used to it, but our bodies still have a stress reaction every time the dog barks.

When buying appliances, research their noise levels. Even a refrigerator can cause significant noise. Search online for "noise ratings" for the type of appliance you're buying. If you move, look for a place in a quiet area. This is not always easy, as neighbors may change, new dogs come into the neighborhood, and so on. At least you can try to stay away from highways, busy streets, and airports. Avoid schools, churches, stores, and parks, which attract traffic. Before you make the decision to move to a new place, spend time there at different hours of the day and night, weekends and weekdays, to get a sense of the noise level. Talk to the neighbors and ask if anyone has frequent loud parties, band practice, or arguments. We were surprised when we lived far from the airport to discover we were under the landing path of a regular flight that arrived at 4:30 am. Conversely, when we moved a few miles from the airport, we had no air traffic at all.

Outside our homes, we have far less control. Perhaps shutting windows can make a difference. One friend installed a new, triple-pane window so that she couldn't hear her new neighbors yelling at each other.

You can combine choosing silence with almost all of the other techniques, including breathing, smiling, loving, gratitude, affirmations, forgiveness, and prayer.

When to:

Think about something you can do to choose silence at home or work. You can affirm right now, "The next time I _____, I will choose silence."

Visualize

Studies show that visualizations can increase motivation, confidence, attention, planning, and memory. Visualizing a physical performance, such as in athletics, music, theater, or speaking, improves performance, motor control, perception, strength, power, coordination, and agility. Visualizing yourself as loving, grateful, forgiving, and calm can help you achieve those qualities.

You can visualize almost anywhere, anytime. The best time may be as you first wake up or right before you go to sleep, as this is when your subconscious is most receptive.

I was in Italy one summer on business. The morning I got to the airport to return home, I realized I did not have a seat assignment. Since I was alone and it was peak travel season, chances were high that I would be assigned a middle seat in the back. Rather than worrying about it, I was in a good mood. It was a long line, moving slowly, yet I was happy and relaxed. After a while, I started breathing and visualizing love flowing into me and from me. When I finally got to the clerk, she was happy to see me, and I was happy to see her. We chatted about Italy and Hawaii and wished each other a good day. I didn't even check my boarding pass. When I boarded the plane and started to turn right down the aisle, the flight attendant pointed to the left and said I was in first class. The clerk had upgraded me from Italy to England and then on to Los Angeles!

Other times, I have visualized love to make a line move faster, and it didn't work. When I was in Italy, I did not visualize love to get something. That's why it worked—it came from a pure heart.

How to:
There are at least three types of visualizations.

Visualize physical activity: Olympic athletes use visualizations to train their brains for performance. You can too, whether you are an athlete, musician, or want to improve your performance at work such as running a meeting, selling to a client, coaching an employee, or giving a presentation.

Use detailed, vivid images to rehearse the entire performance mentally. Engage all the senses to set the scene: see who is there, feel your positive emotions, hear what is around you, smell the air, see your clothes and equipment. Imagine yourself arriving, performing, and finishing with success. Research shows that athletes who visualize perform better than those who do not. By the way, they do not visualize winning itself. Instead, they visualize the elements of an excellent performance.

Visualize a positive future: Self-help books like *The Secret* say that you can achieve health and wealth if you visualize yourself healthy and wealthy. Many people say this has worked for them. They might make a prosperity board with pictures of the car they want to drive, the house they want to buy, the clothes they will wear, and so on. They combine these visualizations with affirmations, such as "I am healthy, I am wealthy." The great motivational speaker Jim Rohn had this caution: "Affirmation without action is delusion." There is some research suggesting that these types of visualizations and affirmations are not effective. Instead, studies have found that what works is questions. Rather than saying to ourselves, "I am wealthy" which the subconscious might reject and even sabotage, we can ask, "How will I be wealthy?" This may free the subconscious mind to figure out ways to become wealthy. Then you can visualize the specific steps to achieve wealth, and act on them.

Visualize love: As you breathe in, visualize love flowing into your heart. As you breathe out, visualize love flowing from your heart. You can visualize love flowing out to a loved one, your family, co-workers, neighbors, people nearby, community, and the world.

You can combine visualizing with many other techniques, including breathing, smiling, loving, gratitude, affirmations, forgiveness, and prayer.

When to:

Think about something you regularly do where you can multitask by visualizing. Is it before you fall asleep, when first waking, or some other time? You can affirm right now, "The next time I _____, I will visualize."

Fast every morning

We've all heard that breakfast is the most important meal of the day, yet recent animal studies have shown that daily, short periods of fasting improved memory and actually grew new brain cells. That's why it's in the section for mental wellness.

When my MD told me about this, I thought he was crazy. He suggested I not eat from about 8 p.m. the night before until about 11 a.m. or noon the next day. He said coffee or tea are okay, and lots of water is essential. I'll admit that the first few weeks all I could think about was food. Even now, after fasting every morning for more than a year, there are still times when I am ready for lunch at 9:30.

I also can testify that my memory has improved dramatically. For years before I started this practice, I could not remember people's names or even faces. It was interfering with my work and social life. After about six months of morning fasting, I noticed a big difference.

Like everything else in this book, if this doesn't appeal to you, go on to something else. There are many reasons not to do this, as explained below. One great benefit of morning fasting is it saves the time and money of preparing breakfast, so it's even better than multitasking.

How to:

There are many different approaches to daily fasting that you can look up online.

In animal studies, daily fasting was associated with longer lifespans and resulted in losing weight. Although human studies are still being conducted and the evidence is not conclusive, daily fasting may have potential benefits for preventing or possibly reversing cancer, inflammation, hypertension, asthma, rheumatoid arthritis, and metabolic syndrome.

The bad news is that fasting also may increase blood pressure and cholesterol levels. Not everyone loses weight (including me). It may create an unhealthy relationship with food, and can increase stress.

Daily fasting is not recommended for women who are pregnant or breast-feeding, and for people with diabetes. In addition, there has been no research on people who are under 18, over 60, or underweight. Athletes should work with a healthcare provider before daily fasting as it may affect muscle mass and performance.

When to:
Right now, if this appeals to you, make a date with yourself to do some research. Then make an appointment with your health care provider to see if it's right for you.

Mental Wellness

Here are the seven techniques for increasing your mental wellness:

Relax your mind
Listen to positive podcasts, audiobooks, and courses
Repeat positive affirmations
Set goals, and assess progress
Choose silence
Visualize
Fast every morning

Consider adding them to your daily routine. And if you can think of other techniques to relax and energize your mind, add them in, too.

Emotional Well-Being

Emotions. They bring us high, they bring us low. Although we may think of events as causing our emotions, research shows that our emotions shape the way we respond to events. Studies also show that we can shift our emotions intentionally. Here are some ways to create positive emotions while you go about your day.

Listen to music

Upbeat music has been found to increase happiness, mood, immune function, athletic performance, and productivity. Meditative and classical music reduce pain and depression and help you sleep better. With soft music, you eat less. All sorts of music can help you drive better, lower stress, and strengthen learning and memory.

Listening to upbeat music is a great way to get and stay motivated to do chores like cooking, cleaning, and laundry. Some years ago I was working downtown. Parking was a half-mile away. I put together a playlist of up-beat songs from the 60s to today for my walk. Sometimes I would be so energized, I bounced on my toes, danced with shuffle steps, and skipped across the street. I'm sure people thought I was weird, but so what. When I got to work I felt great. Then our office moved, and we parked on site. I switched to listening to music on my drive in, "dancing" in my seat, nodding my head in time to the music, and "playing drums" on the steering wheel. One day I bounced into work and one of my colleagues snapped, "Why are you so happy?" It's the music.

How to:

Get out those old records or CDs. Dust off the ear buds. Try a new station on the radio. Explore Pandora® and Spotify®. Feeling stressed? Relax with the classics. Low energy? Put on some upbeat music. And if you're listening to energizing music while working around the house or garage or walking down the street, go ahead and throw in some dance moves.

You can combine listening to music with many other techniques, including breathing, smiling, singing, loving, gratitude, visualizations, forgiveness, prayer, and awe.

When to:

Think about something you regularly do where you can multitask by listening to music. Is it while doing chores, walking to work, or some other time? You can affirm right now, "The next time I _____, I will listen to music."

Smile

Smiling when you're happy might be natural for you, but for some of us, we forget to tell our faces when we're happy. So one part of this technique is to make sure your happiness shows.

Another part is to smile when you're not particularly happy. That's right, we're talking about fake smiling. Here's why. Research suggests that when you smile, it changes your brain chemistry and actually makes you happier. Studies also show that smiling reduces stress and lowers the heart rate. Smiling increases positive thinking. It improves relationships. Smiling strengthens the body's cells, and boosts your mood, productivity, and creativity.

I'm not suggesting we fake smile to fool anyone. Smiling can be a double-edged sword for women. Many of us have had strange men come up and command us to smile—which in my experience has the opposite effect. Smiling in the workplace possibly could be misconstrued if used during a meeting, or with a boss or a subordinate. Yet you can smile when you're alone in your cubicle or office, especially when working on something routine or unpleasant.

Smiling is my favorite technique in this book because it has transformed my life. I first began consciously smiling as a corporate trainer. During a break in class, a student mentioned it seemed I didn't want people to ask questions because I frowned when they did. I assured him I was frowning in concentration, thinking of an answer, and in fact I loved questions. From then on I put a smile on my face while listening to questions.

When I first moved to Hawaii, I walked down the beach every day with a big grin on my face. Everyone I passed smiled back. Somewhere along the way I stopped smiling, and so did everyone else. More recently, I've realized that I have the dreaded "resting bitch face." As I've matured, things have begun to sag. So I started smiling constantly in order to lift my face and retrain my muscles. I'm smiling as I write this. Most of the time when I'm with others, they're not even aware that I'm smiling because my face just looks neutral. The wonderful benefit is that when

I meet people's eyes, my smile is ready. I smile more often, and they do too—even when I'm walking on the beach.

You can smile pretty much anytime, anywhere. One good time to practice is when you're standing in line. Whether it's at government offices, stores, cafes, restaurants, clubs, theaters, or bathrooms, we spend a lot of time standing in lines. We're probably not too happy about it, which gives you all the more reason to smile. Another time to smile is while listening to someone speak, either one on one or in a group. A small smile can encourage the person speaking that you are listening and even agreeing.

How to:
Experiment with smiling. You can do it right now. Try smiling with a closed mouth, then with an open mouth. You can make it a small smile or a huge grin. It may feel weird at first, but soon it will feel more natural. Keep smiling for the rest of the day, whenever you think of it. Smile wherever you go. Smile whenever you meet someone's eyes.

You can combine smiling with many other techniques, including breathing, loving, gratitude, visualizations, forgiveness, prayer, and awe.

When to:
Think about something you regularly do where you can multitask by smiling. Is it standing in line, sitting at the computer, or some other time? You can affirm right now, "The next time I _____, I will smile."

Sing and chant

The benefit of singing and chanting is that they force deep breathing, which lowers blood pressure. Studies show that singing and chanting are both calming and energizing. They increase happiness and reduce anxiety, stress, and depression. When done in a group, singing and chanting reduce loneliness and enhance feelings of trust and bonding.

I sing whenever I want to get energized or lift a down mood, and always on the way to work. Some of my favorites are oldies like the Beatles "Good Day Sunshine," and James Brown, "I Feel Good;" reggae such as Big Mountain's "Lighten Up," and Michael Franti's "Once a Day;" and pop songs like Hoku Ho's "Perfect Day." For meditative chanting, I love "I Am So Blessed" by Karen Drucker.

I asked my friend Meredith, who has four young children, about how she uses singing while driving with the kids. Here's what she said.

> It is important to me that my children feel like music can help them express their interior life, and that they feel they can let loose and belt out a song. It's been about a year since I started singing with them in the car, and I find that drives are a lot less stressful—whenever they start fighting in the car, I just play their song list and everyone sings the whole time. Not just less stressful: happy. We have about 30 songs on the list, and I add and take out a couple to mix things up every six weeks or so.
>
> I created a playlist based on a bunch of criteria that I deemed important:
>
> -Foundational songs or groups (for us, that is Erasure, the Beatles, Abba, Cat Stevens, A Tribe Called Quest, Queen, Indigo Girls)
>
> -A couple of their picks ("Roar," "Life's a Happy Song," "Shut up and Dance")
>
> -Songs that are punny, funny, or make them think ("Rhode Island is Famous for You," "If I Had $1,000,000," "Please be a Ninja")

-Songs that celebrate ("Once a Day," "Can't Keep it In," "I Like it that Way," "Lovely, Love my Family")

-Songs with harmonies and different rhythms ("Tell me something Good," "Cassiopeia," "Power of Two," "Up Up Up," "Pata Pata")

-And most of all, songs that are fun to sing ("Cups," "Good Morning Baltimore," "Somebody to Love," "Twist and Shout").

I love hearing their chirpy little voices singing around the house, and it's an easy way to see how a seed you plant in a child's brain can bloom. That is one way I have made their lives better.

Because of the nature of the songs I pick, the topics can spur conversation or ideas. As they get older, it becomes increasingly important to have as many inroads as possible to connect and communicate with them in different ways. I feel closer to them, and I hope when they grow they remember these times with fondness.

Isn't that wonderful?

How to:
Just sing! Sing on your own, sing karaoke style with musical background, or sing along with your favorite singers. If you've got extra time, join a chorus or choir.

Sing songs that are positive. Positive songs can be found in almost any genre: gospel or other faith songs, show tunes, reggae, oldies, rock, pop, country. Songs can be upbeat and energizing, or relaxing.

If you know Christian, Buddhist, Hindu, Jewish, Hawaiian, or other spiritual chanting, you can chant, too. Chanting can be repeating a mantra aloud, such as "Om namah Shivaya" or "Nam-myoho-renge-kyo," or more complex. Reciting the rosary is a form of chanting. I've used an "Om namah Shivaya" tune and replaced the words with "Peace, health, love, joy, smile." Another chant I made up uses the words "Loving-Kindness."

You can combine singing and chanting with at least two other techniques—breathing and smiling. If you really enunciate your vowels, you can exercise your face, too.

When to:

Think about something you regularly do where you can multitask by singing or chanting. Is it while driving, in the shower, or some other time? You can affirm right now, "The next time I _____, I will sing or chant."

Silently sing or chant

Silent singing and chanting have many of the same benefits as singing and chanting aloud: calming yet energizing, increased pleasure, reduced anxiety, stress, and depression. They engage your lungs and cause relaxation.

I like to sing silently while gardening. It allows me to listen to the birds and the breeze while still getting the benefit of singing.

You can silently sing or chant while doing laundry, gardening, and other household tasks. Perhaps you can do it at work. If you're shy about singing aloud while driving with your family, this might be a good alternative for you. You can do it whenever you don't want to be heard, but can still move your lips.

How to:

How do you silently sing or chant? You move your lips and tongue as you would normally. Rather than vocalizing, breathe out the words. You can say the words in a whisper, or completely silently. Try it now. Notice how it still involves deep breathing.

The songs you silently sing can be the same uplifting and inspiring ones as you would sing aloud.

You can combine silent singing and chanting with at least one other technique—smiling.

When to:

Think about something you regularly do where you can multitask by silently singing or chanting. Could it be while doing chores, gardening, or something else? You can affirm right now, "The next time I _____, I will silently sing or chant."

Laugh

Laughing increases happiness and relaxation, and improves sleep. It strengthens the immune system and boosts energy. Laughter reduces pain and stress. It even lowers blood sugar levels.

In his memoir, *Anatomy of an Illness*, Norman Cousins wrote about the pain and sleeplessness he had as a result of a disabling spine condition. He found that watching the Marx Brothers and Candid Camera helped him feel better, reduce pain, and get to sleep.

I am a huge fan of comedy and have tried my hand at both improv and standup. As a speaker and trainer, I love to get people laughing and to laugh with them. I enjoy making people laugh in conversation and on the street. When you make people laugh and laugh with them, you all feel good.

Many of the training programs I present are on HR law compliance for managers, and harassment prevention for employees. So don't tell me that your work is too serious for laughter. You can have fun no matter what your job. I have been at funerals where we all cried because we were laughing so hard. Of course, humor has to be done right. I don't believe in telling jokes. Instead, see the funny side of the situation.

I also practice laughter yoga on the drive to important meetings and before making presentations. It lifts my energy and mood and makes it more likely that I will be funny and make them laugh. I've taught laughter yoga in my stress reduction and body yoga classes. After we all have laughed for a few minutes, we end up giggling and guffawing for the rest of the class. Everything just looks funnier. Many students say it is the high point of the class for them.

Driving to work is a great time to laugh. According to the U.S. Census, about 76% of us commute to work in our cars alone. Average commute one way is 25 minutes, so that's almost an hour a day. Many people use this precious time to listen to news or talk radio. Others, seeking to be productive, make phone calls for work or family. Some listen to music, while others spend the time worrying about the past or the future. Whatever you do, ask yourself how it makes you feel. By the time you get where you're going, do you feel down, frazzled, or worse?

You can feel relaxed, energized, and happy during your commute by laughing. You can listen to comedy while driving with the family, too. Laughing together is a great way to bond. And if some family members laugh and others don't, that may be a place to have a meaningful conversation.

Laugh whenever you can, as often as you can.

How to:
When we talk about laughing, we mean roaring with big belly laughs.

Humor in life: hang out with funny people. Make your friends and family laugh. See the funny side of things.

Comedy: find comedians or shows that make you laugh. YouTube,® Pandora,® and SiriusXM® have comedy channels. You'll find the top new comedians and the classics, too, such as George Carlin, Chris Rock, and Joan Rivers. Check out comics and shows from other countries, like the UK and Australia. Even National Public Radio has funny shows and podcasts like *Wait, Wait, Don't Tell Me* and *Car Talk*. If there are improv groups in your area, go to a show. Seek out funny movies and plays.

Laughter yoga: All over the world, people gather together for twenty to thirty minutes a day to practice laughter yoga. You can go online to see how it works, but it's pretty simple. Just laugh! Laugh for no reason. It's fun to do with others, but you can do it all alone.

Laughing naturally involves breathing and smiling, but I don't think laughing can be combined with any other technique in this book! It's a full experience in itself, engaging your body, mind, heart, and spirit.

When to:

Think about something you regularly do where you can multitask by laughing. Could it be while driving or some other time? You can affirm right now, "The next time I _____, I will laugh."

Love your work

Love your job. If you can't love all of it, love some of it. If you can't love the work, love the way you do your work. Or just love your colleagues.

When we don't love our work, we feel stressed, which can cause health problems. When you love what you do, you feel energized, happy, and productive.

What parts of your job do you love? I asked this of a group of nurses, and after an uncomfortable silence, one of them said "Lunch!" Another said, "Birthday parties!" I said lunch and birthday parties were great ways to enjoy the company of co-workers, but what parts of their actual work did they love. Silence. What part of their jobs had they ever loved? Why did they become nurses? One finally said she used to love to give patients neck and shoulder rubs. I asked, "When was the last time you did that?" She said it was years ago. She decided there and then to spend ten minutes a day giving massage. She told me later that it made a huge difference for her. She did it during the afternoon when she was usually low energy. Knowing she was going to do it made her morning go better. While she was giving massage, she enjoyed it. The rest of the day was better because she remembered how much fun she had. Of course, her patients enjoyed it, too. And she noticed after they received massage, they stopped using the call button as frequently—which freed up more time for her to do more massage.

In my seminars, I've asked thousands of people what they love about their jobs. Many answer, "Helping people." If that's true for you, be sure to spend time each day helping people. Savor it while you're doing it. Remind yourself, "I'm helping someone!" Then remember what you achieved as you commute home. I write down my achievements at work to remind myself of my successes.

Another way to love your work is to improve your relationships with co-workers and bosses. Acknowledge them. Where I used to work, on Fridays we took turns cleaning out the refrigerators. The person of the day would send an email to everyone around 3:00 reminding them to label or remove items so they wouldn't get thrown away. Most people didn't acknowledge the email, while others always sent one back thanking them for doing the job, maybe saying something light or humorous to make them feel good.

Our attitude about our work can make all the difference. I had a job with a great boss and colleague, doing work I loved doing, but I got frustrated with things that were out of our control. I left that job but went back after a year. This time, I had a lot more fun because anything that was out of my control I just let go. I could even laugh!

How to:
Remind yourself every day that you are blessed or lucky to have a job.

Whatever you love about your work, plan to do as much as you can every day. Look forward to it, savor it while you are doing it, and then remind yourself of how good it felt the rest of the day.

Build up your relationships with co-workers. How can you make them feel more valued? Perhaps you can ask for their opinion, or thank them for something they've done or said they would do. Forgive them (in your own mind) for the past and the future.

Let go of anything you can't control.

You can combine loving your work with many other techniques, including breathing, smiling, positive affirmations, gratitude, and forgiveness.

When to:
You can affirm right now, "The next time I go to work, I will love _____."

Be grateful

Feeling gratitude improves sleep, resilience, and self-esteem. It increases happiness, empathy, and feelings of health. Gratitude actually increases the likelihood you will exercise and get check-ups. It reduces stress, envy, depression, aggression, resentment, frustration, regret, and trauma.

My husband's family practices gratitude all the time. They thank each other for the smallest things—taking out the rubbish, washing the dishes, doing the laundry—all things they are "supposed" to do. Yet how wonderful it feels to be thanked for doing them.

About a year ago, I started posting three things I was grateful for every day on Facebook. I wasn't doing it for others, though sometimes I tagged a friend I was grateful for seeing that day. I chose to do it on Facebook because I was there already, so it didn't seem like a separate chore. The practice is to pick three different things every day. Some days I really have to think hard to come up with three new things, other days I'm overflowing. It has changed the way I look at the world. On the days when family members or celebrities who affected my life have died, I write all the things about them I appreciated. If I get to the afternoon and don't have anything yet, I start looking for things to be grateful for. I'll call a friend, or go for a walk. Once I spent the whole day doing a deep clean of the house, and when I was completely exhausted the thought popped into my head, "I am grateful I have a house to clean." I've also noticed trends—I love sunrises and sunsets—and being a bit of an introvert, initially my posts were rarely about people. That motivated me to reach out to others more often. This practice has changed my life. And friends have told me that it has made them more grateful, too.

Gratitude is the perfect antidote for jobs which are less than fulfilling. Express gratitude that you are alive, you are healthy enough to be at work, and you have a job. Be grateful for your organization, your bosses, and your co-workers. Be grateful for meetings. Appreciate that the people there included you in this meeting. Be grateful for good things that happen while you are at work, whether a conversation, an accomplishment, or a funny moment. I used to work in a place where the bathrooms often malfunctioned. We were all grateful when they were fixed! Thank the people around you. Thank co-workers for doing their jobs. Thank your boss for being a manager.

Develop a gratitude practice with your family. Go around and have everyone say one thing they are grateful for. To make it fun, everyone has to say something different. A teacher of Hawaiian tradition, Allen Alapai, says that when he was growing up, the family got together every evening and they would each say something they were grateful for, starting with his grandmother. He learned so much about her, his parents, and siblings hearing about what made them grateful that day. After everyone had said what they were grateful for, anyone who was mad at another family member had to forgive them. (See the next section on Forgiveness.)

How to:
Express gratitude from the moment you wake up, because you have another day to live, to the moment you lie down, for all the blessings you experienced that day. Whenever you see something beautiful, you can say, either silently or aloud, "I'm grateful for that (beautiful tree, flower, cloud, mountain, lake, rainbow, sunrise, sunset, baby, kitten, puppy ...)."

If you are a person of faith, you can say "Thank you, God, for this beautiful ..."

Express gratitude to the people all around you. You can thank clerks and waiters, family members for doing their chores, co-workers for just doing their jobs.

At the end of the day, you can write down or just think about three things you are grateful for that day. They should be specific and unique to that day. You can be grateful for a sunrise, a conversation, an accomplishment, an idea, or any other big or small thing that made your day a blessing.

You can combine being grateful with many other techniques, including breathing, smiling, and loving.

When to:

Think about something you regularly do where you can multitask by being grateful. Is it when you're with your family, co-workers, on waking, or at other times? You can affirm right now, "The next time I _____, I will express my gratitude."

Forgive

Forgiveness creates healthier relationships. It leads to better sleep. Forgiveness decreases anxiety, blood pressure, and depression. It improves the immune system, heart health, and psychological well-being. Most importantly, forgiveness increases feelings of spiritual peace.

The first time I practiced forgiveness was a fluke. I had sold my law practice but kept five bad debts. My assistant had been sending bills to these former clients for years trying to get them to pay. The first month after selling the practice, I sent them bills as well. Nothing happened. The second month I printed out the bills again. As I was getting ready to mail them I thought, "This is ridiculous!" Instead of sending them, I wrote on each one, "I forgive you," and put them away in the files. I never contacted the clients again, yet within one month, two of them paid their bills!

A friend of mine was under the mistaken belief that I had done something which hurt him. He was angry and started yelling at me. I tried to get a word in, yet couldn't, so listened silently. Suddenly I thought I should forgive him. I started silently saying, "I forgive you," over and over. In the middle of a sentence he stopped, said, "I don't know why I'm yelling at you, you didn't even do it," and apologized.

Of course, we can't forgive with the intention to get someone to do something. You have to do it for its own sake.

We can practice forgiveness almost anytime, anywhere. One time we can practice forgiveness is when we're stuck in a boring meeting, conversation, speech, or sermon. Start by forgiving the people who put you in the situation. If your boss or spouse made you go, forgive them. If you put yourself in this situation, forgive yourself. Forgive the person speaking who is boring you. Or if it's an important meeting called to deal with a crisis, forgive the people inside the room or outside the room who may be creating the challenges you are discussing.

Then forgive everyone else you can think of to forgive.

If you're on hold on the phone or in an online chat with customer service, decide to forgive the person if they can't help you. Forgive the people who set up the system in such a way that you can't be helped, or that you had to call in the first place.

Develop a forgiveness practice with your family. Everyone gets to name one person they forgive. If the person they forgive is there, that person can thank the other for their forgiveness.

A good time to forgive people is when you're driving. Commit not to yell at or curse other drivers, whether or not they can hear you. I have to admit I used to do that years ago until a friend pointed out that if I ended up dying at that moment, the last words on my lips would be blasphemy.

How to:

How do you forgive the unforgivable? You forgive the people, not their acts. They don't have to know you've forgiven them. You do not forgive them for their benefit, but for yours.

You can say silently to yourself, over and over, "I forgive you." If someone cuts you off in traffic, say "I forgive you." If a family member or someone at work irritates you, think "I forgive you." If the clerk seems unusually slow, remember "I forgive you." If you get an email or see a post that angers you, "I forgive you."

You also can say "I forgive you" out loud to someone who has offended you.

For long-standing grudges, it may take a little more time. For more serious actions, Dr. Fred Luskin in his book *Forgive for Good*, gives a nine-step process for forgiving. I highly recommend this.

You can combine forgiving with many other techniques, including breathing, smiling, and loving.

When to:

Think about something you regularly do where you can multitask by forgiving. You can affirm right now, "The next time I _____, I will practice forgiveness."

Love

The research is overwhelming. The best way to live a long and happy life is to have good relationships. That's not necessarily relationships with a capital R. Although being in a stable long-term marriage is correlated with good health, every time you interact with another person in a positive way you literally are doing good things for your heart.

Loving others enhances not only heart health but also mental health and happiness. It reduces stress and pain. When we love, it decreases blood pressure and prevents chronic illness. We sleep better and live longer.

The more we love, the more we live.

In the book *Man's Search for Meaning*, Viktor Frankl writes that he understood the importance of love in a new way when he was imprisoned as a Jew in a Nazi death camp. One day, the image of his wife came to him. He could see her in every detail. From that day forward, he pictured her and imagined long conversations with her. These images and conversations helped him get through his ordeal. He wrote, "A man who has nothing left in this world still may know bliss, be it only for a brief moment, in the contemplation of his beloved."

A friend who was married to a wonderful man told me they had divorced. I asked what happened. She said he argued about trivial things, such as how the cups and saucers should be stored in the cupboards. It wasn't the appropriate time to say anything, but I thought, "It takes two to have that argument!" A few years later she introduced me to a fabulous man she was dating. Some months after that, she said they had broken up because of an argument. Her other friends were taking sides as to who was right. I said it doesn't matter who was right. Go to him and apologize. Tell him you love him. Forgive him. She did, they are still together, and she recently thanked me for changing her life.

Relationships are so important, they are almost literally a matter of life and death. No one is perfect, including you. Cherish your loved ones.

For many years, I have silently repeated the mantra, "Loving Kindness." One day my husband and I were having a "discussion" about his business. He's an artist and I'm a lawyer, so we have different perspectives, to put it mildly. While he was making his point, I decided to start silently repeating "Loving Kindness." After a few moments, he suddenly came up with another idea that was better than either of the ones we had been arguing for.

Of course, we can't silently repeat "Loving Kindness" with the intention to make people do what we want. I've tried it, and it doesn't work that way.

Make love a family activity. When together as a family, everyone gets to name one person they love, inside or outside the family, and one thing they love about them. To make it fun, each person has to name a different person.

A good time to practice love is on social media. Social media can be good. We can laugh at funny videos. We can be inspired by nature photos and uplifting quotes. We can cry with tears of joy and empathy at the courage and kindness of people all over the world.

Social media also can expose us to everything that is wrong in the world. We can see the worst of people. We can get angry about wrongs and injustices, and feel powerless to do anything about them.

Because it brings out the best and worst of us, social media is a great place to practice love. Send loving thoughts to the people whose posts you read, and the people being posted about. Is someone sick? Send love. Is someone happy? Send love. Someone does something you don't like? Send love. Someone says something you disagree with? Send love.

This is not easy. I'm not even sure it's possible, since I've never achieved it for more than a few minutes at a time. It's something I'm aiming for.

If there are people you often disagree with, another approach is to send them love while you click on the link to unfollow or unfriend them.

In addition to sending love to everyone, be loving in your posts. Give people the benefit of the doubt. See things from their point of view. Don't demonize them as evil or stupid. Almost everyone is rational based on their background and experience.

Post the way you would talk to them if they were with you in person. Or don't post at all. Not everything has to be responded to. Just love.

How to:

Remember love: Think of all of the people in your life who you love, now or in the past. Remember sweet times you had together. Picture them, and send them your love. Think, "I love you!"

Be loving with loved ones: Sometimes it's hard to be loving to loved ones. We can get caught up in the rush of life and barely acknowledge them. They can be irritating—or worse. Yet you love them. Keep love in your voice. Respect them and their ideas. Know they aren't perfect, and neither are you.

Listen with full attention. Hear what they may not be saying. Listen for their emotions. Show your respect and empathy.

Speak positively. Talk about your blessings. Express gratitude and appreciation for them and the beauty in the world. Don't complain. For some of us, this may feel pretty much impossible, yet even one less complaint a day is progress.

Love and forgive. Apologize for misunderstandings and arguments, no matter who started it.

When you touch a loved one, be gentle. If you comb your child's or parent's hair in the morning, you can make your touch gentle and loving, lightly massage the head for a few seconds, and have a fun conversation.

Love others the way they want to be loved. In the mega-best-selling book, *The Five Love Languages*, Gary Chapman identifies five different ways people feel loved: words of affirmation ("I love you," compliments), spending quality time together (hanging out, traveling), acts of service for each other (cooking, fixing things around the house), receiving gifts (flower from the garden, bringing home a special treat), and physical touch (hugs and kisses). If we have a different love language than our partners, they will not feel loved even though we are showing love in our language. My husband, for example, loves to receive gifts. I don't really like gifts; my love language is acts of service. He has spent hours making me a gift when what I really wanted was for him to take on my "honey do" list. Understanding these differences helps me realize he is showing me his love in his way, and gives me the language to express how I want to be loved. I highly recommend this book.

Love everyone: We are all on this earth together. Every person you meet is part of your life. Clerks, waiters, drivers, co-workers, neighbors, and people all over the world want what you want: to be happy, loved, respected. Love them. Respect them. Look kindly into their eyes. Smile. Say a kind word. Speak with a gentle, loving tone of voice. Have a conversation. Talking with another can relax both of you, reducing the heart rate and blood pressure. Show your compassion. Build them up. Compliment them sincerely. They feel better and so do you.

If you're on hold with customer service on the phone or online chat, you're going to be dealing with a real person soon. That person may or may not be able to help you get what you want, yet you can set a goal for the quality of the interaction you have with them. Do you want it to be pleasant? Do you want both of you actually to have fun and enjoy your time together? You can make that happen, with love.

Think love: Remind yourself every day of all the qualities of the ones you love, rather than dwelling on behavior you don't like so much. When a loved one does something you don't like, think love. Send them loving thoughts. Think, "I love you!" Repeat it over and over. Think "Loving-Kindness" wherever you are, all the time.

You can combine being loving with many other techniques, including breathing, smiling, being grateful, and practicing forgiveness.

When to:

Think about something you regularly do where you can multitask by loving others. You can affirm right now, "The next time I _____, I will show love."

Emotional Well-being

Here are the nine techniques for increasing your emotional well-being:

Listen to music
Smile
Sing and chant
Silently sing or chant
Laugh
Love your work
Be grateful
Forgive
Love

Consider adding them to your daily routine. And if you can think of other emotionally uplifting exercises you can do with Mindful Multitasking, add them in, too.

Spiritual Being

Spiritual health has been defined many ways. Some say it is about values, morals, and beliefs. Others say it is having purpose and meaning in our lives. Here, I am using it in the sense of our awareness of something greater than ourselves. You may call that something a Higher Power, the Universe, Spirit, or God. Often we get so wrapped up in ourselves that we forget there is something greater than us. The techniques in this section are designed to quiet the mind, to create a space to see the greatness of the universe, and listen for the still small voice.

Experience awe

When we experience awe, it inspires hope, appreciation, gratitude, and creativity. Awe increases feelings of trust, empathy, generosity, and connection with others. Awe reduces the feeling of being rushed and instills a sense of peacefulness.

What is awe? Anytime you connect with nature and say "Wow!" or "Ahhh," you are in awe.

I used to live on the California coast, two hours south of San Francisco, where I often had business. To get there, I usually took the main highways through the heart of Silicon Valley. A friend suggested that instead, I take the road through open fields along the ocean. Though it took twenty minutes longer, it was awe-inspiring. I always arrived feeling refreshed and rejuvenated, and my work would be excellent as a result.

You don't have to live in California or Hawaii to find awe. Viktor Frankl wrote of the insights he gained imprisoned as a Jew in a Nazi death camp:

> "One evening, when we were already resting on the floor of our hut, dead tired, soup bowls in hand, a fellow prisoner rushed in and asked us to run out to the assembly grounds and see the wonderful sunset. Standing outside we saw sinister clouds glowing in the west and the whole sky alive with clouds of ever-changing shapes and colors, from steel blue to blood red. The desolate grey mud huts provided a sharp contrast, while the puddles on the muddy ground reflected the glowing sky. Then, after minutes of moving silence, one prisoner said to another, "How beautiful the world *could* be!"

Although being outside in nature is the best way to experience awe, even seeing pictures or watching video of nature scenes can engender awe.

How to:
Awe is all around you and takes no extra time to enjoy. Just look up.

You're walking from the car, bus, or train to work, home, or a store. You're walking from work to a lunch spot, or from one building to the next. You're at home, taking out the rubbish.

Every time you go outside, look to the sky. It can be a sunrise, sunset, the moon, clouds, stars, rain, rainbows, the color of the sky, or anything else that touches your soul with the vastness of the universe. Look for the patterns of trees against the sky, the vivid colors of leaves, and the delicate blossoms of flowers. Notice the birds and other wildlife around you.

At home, in the office, or while driving, look up out the windows.

When you see an awe-inspiring sight, stop for a few seconds. Take a deep breath. Savor it. Be grateful. Smile. Enjoy.

When to:
Think about something you regularly do where you can multitask by experiencing awe. Is it while walking, driving, or another time? You can affirm right now, "The next time I _____, I will look to be awe inspired."

Listen to guided meditation

Meditation increases our feelings of peacefulness, well-being, joy, and compassion. It relaxes the muscles. Meditation regenerates brain cells, improving memory, attention, and learning. It decreases stress, inflammation, and pain, and improves our immune function.

For years I have used a twelve-minute guided meditation originally developed by Hans Selye, M.D., the physician who discovered in the 1930s how stress impacts our health. I have it on my phone to use whenever I want, and on an iPod Shuffle® I keep under my pillow. The Shuffle® is ideal because it's tiny and can be operated in the dark just by feel.

You can listen to guided meditation when riding (not driving) in a car, or while sitting and waiting. One of my favorite times to use it was when I was taking the bus to work. Half way through the meditation my shoulders relaxed and my head started nodding, yet I was completely aware of everything around me. (Having said that, if you do use it on public transit, make sure to have your bag on your lap with your arms looped through the handles.)

The time right before you go to sleep is unique and special. Often our last thoughts can make the difference between having a peaceful and restful night, or not. That's why it's a great time to listen to guided meditation. You also can follow guided meditation if you wake up in the middle of the night.

How to:

There are hundreds if not thousands of guided meditations online, in apps, and in CDs, many of them free. Some are designed specifically to induce sleep, others to both relax and energize you. These latter are great for times when you're not in bed. Download one or more to your phone or device. Experiment with different ones until you find the right ones for you.

Put on headphones or earbuds. Sit in a comfortable chair, or lie down on the floor or in bed. Close your eyes, listen, and follow the instructions. Relax.

When to:

Think about something you regularly do where you can multitask by listening to guided meditation. Can it be on going to bed or some other time? You can affirm right now, "The next time I _____, I will listen to guided meditation."

Repeat mantras

A mantra is one or a few words or sounds repeated while meditating, or while going about daily activities. It can be said aloud or silently.

Probably the best-known mantra is the Sanskrit word, "Om," considered in Hinduism to be the most sacred sound. Other mantras include Soka Gakkai's "Nam-myoho-renge-kyo," an expression to manifest the Buddha nature. In Christian tradition, mystics repeat the names "Jesus" and "God."

Although mantras often are taught as sounds with universal meaning, because they are not in English they may be off-putting to some people. However, a mantra can also be a word or phrase in your own language, such as Joy, Peace, or Loving-Kindness.

Repeating a mantra stills the mind. It reduces negative thinking and develops mindfulness. It allows us to become more attentive and present. It enhances our feelings of love and connection to Spirit.

When I was in yoga school at a Hindu temple in Colorado, we learned the mantra, "Om namah Shivaya," honoring the deity Shiva. Although I chanted this along with my fellow students and teachers, on my own time I repeated "Loving-Kindness," because it reminded me of how I wanted to be in every moment. I have chanted Loving-Kindness in the decades since then, and though I still am not perfect, I am making progress.

About a year after graduating from yoga school, I met up with some of the other alums in Hawaii to go swimming with dolphins. We got to the beach and could see them a few hundred yards off shore. We swam out but didn't see anything for 10 minutes. Suddenly, it occurred to me to silently repeat the mantra, "Om namah Shivaya." As soon as I started, the dolphins appeared, and for the next hour they swam next to us, below us, and even jumped over us. When we finally got back to the beach, we compared notes and discovered that one person started the mantra, and then the rest of us picked up on it—as did the dolphins! Incidentally, from this experience I learned that we don't swim with dolphins—dolphins swim with us.

I was in Australia as a guest speaker at a workshop with a Hawaiian elder teacher. One of the students—who had been introduced to the Hawaiian culture a few years before and knew nothing of the language—was going on and on about how the Hawaiian language is sacred. She was taken aback when I blurted in exasperation, "ALL languages are sacred! English is sacred. It's not the language, it's the meaning. Spirit, God, Love. Those words are sacred in every language. And I think they're more sacred for you if they're in your native tongue, because you understand them in the deepest possible way." That's why I prefer mantras in English. But if a mantra in another language appeals to you, use that.

You can repeat a mantra almost anywhere, any time that you don't have to listen for information. One of the times I like to do it is while cooking. When it comes to cooking, there are two types of people. Some love to cook, and they pour their love into their food. Then there are the rest of us. For us, cooking can seem like a chore, and our food may reflect that. That's why cooking is a good time to repeat a mantra. When I do, I enjoy cooking more, and my food tastes better.

Another time to repeat mantras is when in meetings. You can silently repeat "peace," "love," "gratitude," or any other word that may help you in the situation.

How to:
Pick a word or phrase that connects you with others and with Spirit. Repeat it silently or aloud, over and over and over.

You can combine repeating a mantra with other techniques, including breathing and smiling.

When to:

Think about something you regularly do where you can multitask by repeating a mantra. Is it while doing chores, cooking, in meetings, or some other time? You can affirm right now, "The next time I _____, I will repeat a mantra."

Meditate

Unlike guided meditation, discussed above, the meditation we are talking about here is done on your own, without listening to a voice guiding you. The benefits of regular meditation have been proven in hundreds of research studies. Meditation increases feelings of peacefulness, well-being, joy, and compassion. It relaxes muscles. Meditation can actually regenerate brain cells, improving memory, attention, and learning. It decreases stress, pain, and inflammation, and boosts the immune system to prevent disease.

Usually, we think of meditation as sitting with closed eyes. You can do that and it's great, although it does take fifteen or twenty minutes a day.

Walking meditation is an ancient practice, and bringing it forward to today we can meditate while driving, sitting in the stands watching our kids practice, cleaning the house, or while doing almost anything else.

One sunny afternoon I was driving towards Berkeley on the San Francisco Bay Bridge, surrounded by rush hour traffic. My co-worker was riding with me. After a long day of work, we weren't talking, so I meditated while driving. I found myself in perfect sync with the other cars. I seemed to know exactly when to speed up and when to slow down, when to change lanes and when to stay put. As we left the bridge my friend said, "I don't think you hit the brakes once! It was like we were flowing down a river."

Since you shower or bathe every day, that is a great time to meditate. Creative people sometimes say they get their best ideas while showering, and they don't want to lose that opportunity by meditating in the shower. In my experience, you will get more and better ideas when you combine showering with meditation.

How to:

The essence of meditation is stilling the mind and breathing. Some forms of meditation involve stilling the mind by paying attention to the breath. See the section on Breathing for various techniques. Other forms of meditation involve breathing and stilling the mind using a mantra. See the section on Mantras.

When to:

Think about something you regularly do where you can multitask by meditating. Is it while driving, waiting, showering, or some other time? You can affirm right now, "The next time I _____, I will meditate."

Pray

Research has been done on the effects of prayer in many religious traditions. Studies show that prayer reduces stress, blood pressure, use of alcohol, and aggression. Prayer increases relaxation, alertness, trust, forgiveness, self-control, peace of mind, well-being, and joy. It helps you maintain a positive attitude, deal successfully with challenges, and recover more quickly from illness and injury. Prayer boosts the immune system, lessens the severity and frequency of illness, and helps you live longer.

If prayer doesn't appeal to you, go on to the next section.

When I learned the art of ancient Hawaiian massage, called lomilomi (pronounced low-me-low-me), my teacher Auntie Margaret Machado taught us that it is praying work. As a Christian, she taught us always to pray before putting our hands on the patient. After I graduated, I worked as a massage therapist giving foot massage. Usually, I began by silently thanking God for allowing me to be of service to the person, and asking Him to guide my hands. One day a woman came in whose feet were covered with giant blisters. Her skin was taut over the liquid. My first reaction was, "Oh my God!" Clearly I could not give her the usual deep, vigorous foot rub. My next thought was to pray. "Oh God, help me!" I sat down at her feet and heard a voice inside me say, "Just love her feet." Then I remembered the story of Mary Magdalene washing the feet of Jesus. I bathed each foot as if it was a fragile baby, and gently stroked them with lotion. She relaxed and fell asleep. And I was transformed.

I like to start every prayer with "Thank you, God!" Then I thank Him for every good thing I can think of. I keep a prayer book of people I want to remember to pray for.

A good time to pray is whenever we hear or see the news. Television's Mister Rogers said:

> When I was a boy and I would see scary things in the news, my mother would say to me, "Look for the helpers. You will always find people who are helping." To this day, especially in times of

"disaster," I remember my mother's words and I am always comforted by realizing that there are still so many helpers – so many caring people in this world.

You can bless or pray for the victims, the helpers, and the journalists reporting the story. Pray for the "bad guys" too. If you are a Christian, remember Jesus said to love your enemies and pray for those who persecute you. You can pray whenever you hear a siren. Pray for all the people involved, victims and responders. If you get an email or see a post about someone in need, you can pray.

Pray for people all around you. If you're on hold on the phone with customer service, pray all goes well on the call. Pray for the person who will help you on the phone. In a meeting, pray for the people there, and for the issue they're discussing. Pray for others who are not there but who are affected by your decisions. Pray for guidance in what you will say during the meeting.

How to:
Author Anne Lamott says there are two kinds of prayer, "Please" and "Thank You."

You can pray for yourself and for others. Some research suggests that praying for others benefits you more than praying for yourself.

The Rev. Dr. Norman Vincent Peale recommended praying the same way you would have a conversation with someone you love and respect. Just pour out your troubles and ask for help. He tells the story of a businessman who decided to treat God as his business partner, talking over all of his ideas and challenges, with great results.

You can combine praying with many other techniques, including breathing, smiling, loving, forgiving, gratitude, and awe.

When to:
Think about something you regularly do where you can multitask by praying. You can affirm right now, "The next time I _____, I will pray."

Listen and watch for answers

When we combine many of these techniques, such as breathing, praying, choosing silence, meditating, and experiencing awe, we may open ourselves to hearing and seeing the answers to our prayers. Although this may sound a little woo-woo, and I have no research to back it up, if you think back, perhaps you can remember a time you've experienced it. Certainly we can find stories of many people who have found this to be true.

About a year ago, my husband and I decided to sell our house. Long before we put it on the market, I started looking for a new home. We prayed every day to sell our house and to find a wonderful home. We had narrowed our search to three areas, and I spent hours looking at homes online, driving by to scope out the neighborhoods, and attending open houses. In six months, we did not find one house that met our criteria.

Our house sold on a Wednesday. Now we really needed to find a place. The following Saturday, we were running some errands, and I decided to check the online listings on my phone. The first house that came up was perfect! It had everything we wanted. Then I saw it was not in our preferred area. Granted, it was only three miles past where we wanted to be, but there was a freeway interchange in between that had a reputation for bad traffic. I decided to forget that house.

The next day at church, the sermon was about listening and watching for the answers to our prayers. As the minister spoke, I wondered. Was God speaking to me when I saw that house on the phone? The minister reminded us that insanity is doing the same thing over and over and expecting different results. Was I insane to keep looking in the same three areas when we hadn't found anything in all that time?

That afternoon, I went to open houses in our preferred neighborhoods, and the houses were decrepit. Finally, I went to look at that other house. It was wonderful! When I walked into the garden, I felt that this was a sacred place.

Before we put in an offer, we tested the traffic, going to the house in the morning so we could go to work from there, and driving there after work. The traffic was lighter than it was going to and from our current home! We made an offer, it was accepted, and here we are.

All because we listened and watched for answers.

When to:
You can affirm right now, "I am open to listening and watching for answers."

Spiritual Being

Here are the six techniques for spiritual being:

Experience awe
Listen to guided meditation
Repeat mantras
Meditate
Pray
Listen and watch for answers

Consider adding them to your daily routine. And if you can think of other spiritually uplifting exercises you can do with Mindful Multitasking, add them in, too.

Creating More Time

The purpose of Mindful Multitasking is to do what you can without taking any extra time. But what could you do if you had a bit more time?

How to make time

How do you create more time?

Reduce screen time. According to the Nielsen Company, in the first three months of 2016, Americans spent an average of 10 hours and 39 minutes A DAY on smartphones, tablets, TV, radio, computers, and video games—not including time at work. It's probably more now.

I am always amused when I read people's posts on Facebook that they are overwhelmed and don't have time. I want to say to them, "Here's a way to get more time: get off Facebook!" One of my students tried this and was astonished at the results. First, he had to admit that though he had limited his kids' screen time, it never occurred to him to limit his own. He decided to reduce his social media from two hours to fifteen minutes a day. He found he didn't miss it at all. In one week he read two and a half novels. It lifted his mood. He felt better. With social media, he got drawn into negativity. With the novel, yes there were negative events, but they weren't real. There was nothing he had to think or do about them.

A woman told me that she stopped watching so much TV and did a jigsaw puzzle instead. She had so much fun doing it, her husband encouraged her to do more. After she had worked on the puzzle for a time, she went to visit a sick friend. She had been dreading seeing him, yet she was so happy from the puzzle that she brought her mood of joy and optimism to the hospital and made him happy.

Reduce screen time, and do something you love instead.

Change birthdays and holidays. If you love to celebrate birthdays and holidays the way you do, that's great. Keep doing it and go on to the next section. However, if your "celebrations" have become chores, if you're dragging yourself through the holidays doing things you are "supposed" to do, here are two ideas. One is to infuse with love everything you do for the birthday or holiday. As I write Christmas cards, I visualize each person and repeat in my mind, "I love you!" While cooking, shopping, and cleaning the house, I keep in mind the people I'm doing it for. Each activity is a gift for my loved ones. The second idea is to consider stopping some (or all) of what you're doing—whether gift giving, cooking, hosting, or something else. Tell your friends and family you can't do it anymore. If someone else feels strongly about it, they can do it. Don't let them guilt you into doing something you don't want to do. Yes, it may be hard, and you may get resistance. On the other hand, maybe they feel the same way and are grateful when we suggest changing our traditions.

Changing our relationship with our kids. I don't have kids, so feel free to ignore my suggestions. I see two common themes among some of my friends. One is where the parents seem to be at the beck and call of the kids. One of my friends called and said she had to cancel our walk because she had to take her 13-year-old son to the store. Why? He wanted a new comic book that had just come out. I'm sorry, that's ridiculous. He can wait until it's convenient for her. Or if he's so desperate, he could take the bus or ride his bike to the store a mile away. The second theme is that the kids don't do anything to help around the house. Though the kids have chores, they don't do them or don't do them right, which leads to a lot of yelling and hand-wringing, though it doesn't get the chores done. At a minimum, in my opinion, kids should be setting and clearing the table, washing the dishes and putting them away, making their beds, folding their laundry, sweeping, vacuuming, and cleaning the bathroom. As they get older, they can make dinner for the family. I've heard people say this is treating kids like servants. No, it's treating kids as equals—equal to you. Because if they don't do it, you will. Family is a team sport. It's more fun for everyone if chores are shared. Not only will you free up more time for yourself, but also your kids will be developing skills they'll need for the rest of their lives. You are actually doing them a favor. I have watched friends who've raised their kids this way, and those kids excelled in school, got great jobs, and married well. They are healthier and happier than the other kids, and their parents are healthier and happier too.

Changing the relationship with our spouse or partner. As long as I'm saying controversial things, I might as well go all the way. I am happily married, so I can speak from experience on this one. One of the qualities that my husband and I love about each other is that we're not "joined at the hip." We have different interests, different friends, different schedules. We often go out together, and we often go out separately. One of us may stay home, working, while the other goes to the gym, for a walk, or to meet friends. This frees up time for him to do his art and for me to do my writing. It also respects the fact that he is an extrovert, and I'm an introvert. For those who sometimes feel they're being dragged to events they don't want to attend, or staying home when they could be doing something out, perhaps this idea will work for them.

Eat less. Another way to create more time is to eat less. Earlier we talked about daily fasting, where we don't eat breakfast. Research also suggests that significantly reducing the overall amount of calories we eat regenerates brain cells and prevents loss of brain function as we get older. You can eat less by simplifying your meals. A quick salad or soup for lunch or dinner may be all you need, and think of all the time you'll save.

Simplify Your Life. That's the name of a book written by Elaine St. James in 1994. There are lots of great ideas in it for making more time for yourself. Its principles inspired my husband and me to move closer to work to save an hour a day, and then to move again to downsize our mortgage so we could retire when we wanted. The book has many easier ideas as well.

What could you do to create more time? Think about your daily or weekly routine. What could you change to get more time to do what you love?

Do what you love

A Native Hawaiian elder once scolded me for working so hard and said, "Life is for delight!" He told me to do what I love to do.

When I teach stress management for busy people, I ask them to think about something they love to do. Most people have to think hard even to remember what they love to do. If they can't remember, I suggest they think about what they loved to do when they were twelve years old. That brings up smiles as they remember the good times. Then when I ask, "When is the last time you did that?" for most people it is years or even decades.

What do you love to do? Here are some of the answers I've heard from students:

- Call or visit a friend or family member
- Play games indoors
- Play games outdoors
- Ride a bike, skate, skateboard
- Play with your pets
- Read for fun
- Write a story, article, poem, song, journal
- Attend movies, plays, shows, concerts
- Visit museums, galleries, beach, park
- Go to festivals, farmers' markets
- Garden
- Sew
- Cook or bake
- Do arts and crafts
- Scrapbook
- Do crossword or jigsaw puzzles
- Sing
- Play music
- Dance
- Walk or hike
- Fly a kite

- Swim or surf
- Take a bubble bath
- Perform in plays, shows
- Watch sunrise, sunset, the stars
- Volunteer
- Make love

What do you love to do?

Make time, and then do it!

Many of my students say this one idea has transformed their lives.

What to do with more time

When you get more time, in addition to doing what you love to do, you also could do some things that you know will give you a healthier, happier life.

1 – 5 minutes

Stretch and exercise.

Take vitamins and supplements. Don't just take supplements because someone said it might be good. It's best to work with a healthcare provider who knows the latest research and who can assess what works for you.

5 – 20 minutes

Stretch and exercise.

Be a good steward of money. Pay your bills. Stay out of debt. It takes time to be a good steward of money, but it takes more time to be broke.

Play with your kids. Go outside and play. Run, jump, and climb. If your child plays sports, you can practice and train with them at home. St. Louis Cardinals baseball manager Mike Matheny had coached his son's Little League team before he got called up to the majors. One of his rules for parents was that they needed to practice throwing a ball with their kids. Whether it's baseball, football, basketball, soccer, boxing, or anything else, practicing or cross-training with your child combines three essentials for both of you: exercising, developing the exercise habit, and building a good relationship.

Meditate. The classic form of meditation is sitting in a chair, or on a pillow on the floor, for 20 minutes in the morning and/or evening. Breathe deeply, and still your mind.

Learn something new. Learning can regenerate brain cells and prevent loss of brain function as we get older. Particularly helpful are learning a new language, playing music, dancing, and exercise. There is virtually no evidence that so-called "brain games" that we can get online actually help brain function.

Keep a health log. If we have chronic illness, difficulty sleeping, problems with elimination, anxiety attacks, or any other disease that may be triggered or worsened by stress, we can start a health log. Write down what time you got up, how your sleep was, note your energy level, everything you eat and drink, any stressful events, exercise, naps, bowel movements, and the time you go to bed. After a while, you may want to create a spreadsheet to see any trends. Take this with you when you see your health care provider so you can answer questions. This has been one of the best things I've ever done to help me understand what's going on with my body.

Take a nap (maybe). When it comes to naps, there are two kinds of people. Some can take a quick nap, wake up feeling great, and be productive the rest of the day. Others are like me. We have a hard time waking up, when we do we feel groggy, and that night we don't sleep well. Figure out what type you are. If naps are good for you, take them. If naps aren't good for you, walk outside for a few minutes, stretch, breathe, put on energizing music, do something fun, or have a conversation.

30 – 60 minutes

Sleep. Most adults need seven to eight hours of sleep. Instead of spending time looking at a screen, go to bed earlier. And if we have difficulty sleeping, we should get away from all screens an hour before bedtime. There is also an app called f.lux which changes the hue of the computer screen after sundown from blue to pink. I've found it helpful for feeling more relaxed at night.

Exercise. If we don't like exercise, how can we get ourselves to do it? My mother, who is now 90, still exercises as she has every day for almost her entire life. Her secret? "Get out of bed, go to the bathroom, put on your exercise clothes, and walk out the door. Don't think! If you think, you'll talk yourself out of it."

Walking is good. If walking in your neighborhood is not interesting, drive to another, or to a park or open space. A good time to do that may be on the way to or from work.

If you want to step it up and get maximum benefit, find an exercise you love to do. Keep trying different things until you find one you love. As a yoga and Pilates teacher, the last thing in the world I thought I would enjoy is boxing, yet I love it.

Increase the likelihood you will exercise by taking classes, exercising with a buddy, or hiring a personal trainer. You can exercise with a buddy virtually—call or text each other when you start your exercise each day. Or become a certified instructor and teach an exercise class. That's how I became a Pilates instructor. I knew it was good for me, and I thought if I taught I would have to do it. There were times I wasn't feeling 100% and would not have gone if I had been taking a class, but since I was teaching I had to go. Once there, I thought that I would just do the first few exercises. Next thing I knew, I had completed the whole class.

Make love. Relationships are the key to a happy, healthy life, and making love keeps relationships happy and healthy too. Sex also can regrow brain cells, and improve mental health, memory, and mood. Aaahhhh.

Research eating right. Eating right is a process. We all know we should eat fresh fruits and vegetables (except people with diabetes have to be careful with fruit, and those on blood thinners have to avoid leafy green vegetables). From there it can get confusing. All of these things are controversial, with some people touting their benefits, and others saying they are unhealthy: fruit juice, vegetable juice, protein shakes, meat, fish, tofu, and pasta. So you need to research, work with your health care provider, experiment, and pay attention to how your body responds.

A good way to begin is to start where you are. If you eat fast food often, go to the company's website and figure out which are the most nutritionally balanced foods they offer. This takes some study. For example, McDonald's site says their nutrition information does not include dressings and sauces. Most salad dressings are fat bombs. You can bring your own light or olive oil dressing, and then add in those calories, fat, sugar, and salt to those in the salad. Another thing you will want to determine is how many calories you should eat at each meal, how much fat, and how many carbs.

I've chosen to follow a Mediterranean diet because there is so much research proving how healthy it is. Sadly, this does not mean I get to eat pasta and pizza every day. It's about eating lots of fruits, vegetables, olives, legumes, and beans. People in other parts of the world eat different recipes with similar ingredients. According to the research reported by the Blue Zones Project of the National Geographic, people live longer, healthier lives in these areas: Ikaria, Greece; Loma Linda, California; Sardinia, Italy; Okinawa, Japan; and Nicoya, Costa Rica. It should be noted, though, that it's not just what they eat, it's how they live their lives—doing almost everything we talk about in this book, including exercise, praying, and having good relationships.

Cook. One of the best ways to use your extra time is to cook at home, using fresh fruits and vegetables. Almost anything you make at home will be healthier than anything from a restaurant.

Use technology to get better. Spire® is a biofeedback device that attaches to your belt or bra, measures the rate of your breathing, and works with your smartphone to alert you when you are not calm. There are other devices made by other manufacturers as well. I found it useful for seeing what activities make me feel calmer.

Superbetter® is a book, website, and app that turns your life into a game. You get points for going on quests, achieving epic wins, working with allies, using power-ups, and fighting the bad guys. Your quests can be anything you want, as big as recovering from PTSD, to as small as cleaning the fridge.

A Mindful Multitasking Manifesto

I am getting fit in no time by:

breathing deeply
tightening my abs
using good body mechanics
relaxing my muscles
rolling my neck & shoulders
exercising my face
extending my back
stretching my hamstrings
standing up and walking around
balancing on one foot
doing squats and lunges
stretching
relaxing my mind
listening to positive podcasts, audiobooks, and courses
repeating positive affirmations
setting goals, and assessing progress
choosing silence
visualizing
fasting every morning
listening to music
smiling
singing and chanting

silently singing or chanting
laughing
loving my work
being grateful
forgiving
loving
experiencing awe
listening to guided meditation
repeating mantras
meditating
praying
listening and watching for answers
doing what I love

Transform Your Life

So that's it! Thirty-four techniques designed to help you achieve physical fitness, mental wellness, emotional well-being, and spiritual being, all through Mindful Multitasking. We also covered some ideas for creating more time in your life, a reminder to use that extra time to do what you love, and suggestions for ways to spend extra time to become even more happy and healthy.

Just implementing a few of these ideas can transform your life. You will live longer, be stronger, think smarter, feel better, and look younger, all while enjoying life and making the world a better place for all the people you meet.

My request to you is that you try it and let me know how it goes. What sounded good? What didn't? What worked? What didn't? What new ideas did you come up with? How can this book be improved? How else can I support you? You can reach me at Makana@MakanaChai.com

Let's share this journey to continue to transform our lives and the world around us.

Thank you – Mahalo

Thank you to everyone who has supported me in this book. Many asked to see an advance copy, which let me know the concept was good.

Dr. Alice Brown gave me many fine suggestions for improvement.

As she has with my last two books, Kumu Brenda Mohalapua Ignacio-Gore has been a guiding light, as well as a great editor.

Thank you to all of the students who took my yoga, Pilates, and stress management classes. You inspired me!

Most of all I want to thank Michael Keolamau Tengan, who was my personal trainer for four years. During those years while we laughed and sweated, we had deep conversations and encouraged each other in our life's paths. His patience and good humor were endless. When he heard about the idea for this book, he would not let me let it go. Mahalo Michael.

About the Author

Makana Risser Chai (born Rita M. Risser) is an attorney and massage therapist. She is certified as a Stress and Wellness Consultant with the Canadian Institute of Stress, and as a facilitator of forgiveness training by the Stanford Forgiveness Project.

She presents programs on Mindful Multitasking, work-life balance, and stress management for people in corporations and associations.

She taught yoga and Pilates for eight years, and is the author of two books on ancient Hawaiian healing massage, one published by the Bishop Museum, the other a winner of the "Keep it Hawai'i" Award.

Before moving to Hawai'i, she wrote a book for Prentice Hall (*Stay Out of Court! The Manager's Guide to Preventing Employee Lawsuits*) and founded a training company based in Silicon Valley to help companies create respectful workplaces. She presented more than a thousand programs on managing within the law and preventing sexual harassment in 38 states for companies such as Oracle and Cisco.

Having lived a stressful life for many years, she developed Mindful Multitasking for busy people who thought they didn't have time to be fit in body, mind, heart, and spirit.